JOHN ANDERSON

The Man Behind the Mask

mcgeary media

First published by McGeary Media 2021

Copyright © 2021 by John Anderson

All rights reserved. No part of this publication may be reproduced, stored or transmitted in any form or by any means, electronic, mechanical, photocopying, recording, scanning, or otherwise without written permission from the publisher. It is illegal to copy this book, post it to a website, or distribute it by any other means without permission.

The Memoir Man
07967 023083
www.thememoirman.co.uk

Second edition

Editing by Michael McGeary

This book was professionally typeset on Reedsy.
Find out more at reedsy.com

Contents

Foreword   iv
Preface   v
1   The Elgan Marvel   1
2   War Baby   7
3   The College   13
4   The Back Story   19
5   Falling for Freda   26
6   Flying High   30
7   In the Line of Fire   36
8   Down to the Bones   43
9   Life in General   47
10   Fishermen and Friends   55
11   Top Doc   61
12   Private Eyes   67
13   To Pastures New   72
14   Hip Service   79
15   Sir John's Legacy   86
16   Joint Responsibility   93
17   Doc Holidays   97
18   Pain in Spain   101
19   A Family Home   106

Foreword

To those who knew John there is little to be said. To those who didn't have the pleasure of him crossing their path, John was without doubt the founder of modern orthopaedics in Middlesbrough.

He had a vision to take The James Cook Hospital to the forefront of modern medicine and also a charisma which attracted colleagues who were themselves of national and international renown to Middlesbrough.

All could have had inspiring careers in prominent posts, but in John they saw something greater and joined him to share the vision.

His patients idolised him and he worked tirelessly to try to help them. Many patients still proudly proclaim that their hip or knee was done by John and you could tell a typical John Anderson signature joint replacement from the x-ray, such was their reproducible standard.

To those who worked with him he was an inspiration and taught to so much to so many. He was a man with a big heart and always remained connected to his Middlesbrough roots. He was a gentleman to all, regardless of title or role, and always had a greeting and a joke.

But, above all, John was a family man and was extremely proud of his children and grandchildren and his passing will leave a chasm in their lives.

So farewell, big John, an inspiration to many, gone but never forgotten.

Andy Port
Chief of Service of Trauma, Orthopaedics, A&E and Theatre Centre, James Cook University Hospital

Preface

John Anderson
January 21st 1941 – August 6 2020

Whenever he phoned me, Dad's greeting was always the same: "How's my lovely favourite daughter?" This made me smile every time – I am, after all, his only daughter, but Dad certainly had a skill for making me and many others feel special.

More than a brilliantly skilled surgeon with a passion for his work, he was also a charismatic man with an excellent bedside manner and always would take his time to explain complicated procedures in layman's terms.

Grateful patients regularly turned up at our door with gifts of cigars, whisky, hampers or a nice bottle of Champagne and genuine, heartfelt thanks.

His passion and work ethic were possibly too much at times. As kids, we accompanied him around the hospital wards on Christmas Day carrying huge sacks full of boxes of biscuits and chocolates to be given out to nurses, porters and switchboard operators as he thanked them all individually.

Importantly, he very much knew he couldn't have achieved all this on his own – his rock was Freda and he loved her by his side.

Dad was a man of principle, an honest man with integrity and professionalism. It is ironic that as his days with the NHS drew to a close, he was diagnosed with diabetic neuropathy, and this along with arthritis and hypotension caused him to gradually become less mobile. He could no longer work at the same speed and do everything he used to do.

Being an "all or nothing" person this frustrated him. However, this did not stop him. He might have had the occasional moan, but he was not one to give in. Indeed, he would do anything to help someone out. We could always rely on Dad.

He was a brilliant grandad and loved spending time with his grandchildren. Nothing was too much trouble and he would travel north and south to watch his grandchildren's sports games. With a houseful of grandkids at Cambridge Road, he was in his element.

He worked hard to ensure that the whole family regularly met up together whether for a meal out or a game of footy. To his grandchildren, he was a friend, a mentor and an inspiration.

Dad was a man of faith, although he never went on about it but just made it part of his daily life, regularly using the phrases "Praise the Lord", "Keep the faith" and when saying goodbye, "If the Lord spares me."

He loved chatting to the local priests and hearing all their stories. On one occasion before operating on a local priest, he held up the surgical instruments and quoted a famous line from Henry II: "Who will rid me of this turbulent priest?"

Although amusing to the operating team at the time, the priest was not quite under the anaesthetic and remembered everything Dad had said.

Dad was a genuine man of the people and loved a good chat and a bit of banter with anyone.

When asked at the palace what he had done to deserve his CBE in 2004, he simply said he hadn't done anything special, he'd just done his job. Indeed, he often said that there was nothing like the feeling of seeing the happiness that a new hip or knee joint gave his patients and the transformation of their lives that followed.

His honesty, integrity, commitment and hard work to the noble cause of medicine are a lesson to us all. He was a gifted man who used his skills to make a difference to the lives of many people in Teesside and we are immensely proud of him.

His guiding light will shine on. He will continue to be part of our lives, right here in our hearts, and he will continue to inspire us.

As Dad would say: "Keep the faith"

Rachael Anderson

1

The Elgan Marvel

It was St George's Day, 1984. I'd been enjoying a fishing break on the River Deveron in Aberdeenshire with my Middlesbrough General Hospital colleagues Dougal Caird and Wray Ellis. As usual, on our regular trips to Scotland, we arranged to meet up just outside Edinburgh, which was halfway back home. We always travelled in our own cars so that if someone had to leave suddenly to deal with an emergency, the other two could stay. Even though it was early spring there was still plenty of snow on the ground, piled high at the sides of the road. I remember coming round a long bend but after that, it all gets a little bit vague. It appears that I lost control as the BMW I'd only had for a few months skidded on a patch of black ice and rolled over. The car only came to a halt when it slammed into a snowbank. I was knocked unconscious by the impact of the crash but could vaguely make out two old ladies flicking through my wallet looking for identification.

"Och look, he's a doctor!" one of them said.

They called for an ambulance and I was taken to Aberdeen Royal Infirmary. When I didn't turn up for the rendezvous, Dougal and Wray knew something was wrong. Dougal rang my wife Freda from a little phone box that I pass now whenever we go up to Edinburgh.

"John hasn't met up with us," he told her. Moments later Freda got a call from the hospital telling her what had happened. She rang Dougal, who immediately got back into his car and drove the two hundred miles back to Aberdeen to see me. That's a real mate, that. I was in hospital for five days and my son Matthew brought Freda up. I had a head injury, but they didn't seem too concerned about that. Most of their attention was being given to my severely mangled finger. An injury like that was pretty bad news for a surgeon. They taped it up but I couldn't operate for six weeks. With work out of the question we headed off to our favourite hotel in Spain, the Los Monteros, just outside Marbella, to chill out for a week. Not long after we got home we found out Freda was pregnant, with Ben, our baby. The other kids pulled our legs, saying we couldn't even be trusted to go away on holiday together!

I soon got back to work but I felt quite strange for a while and could tell something wasn't as it should have been. Almost a quarter of a century would pass, however, before I found out what the problem was. It was 2007, just after I'd retired. I was washing up the dishes after dinner when some fluid ran out of my nose. I also felt some pain, which continued for a couple of days and then got worse. I went to see a colleague, who thought it was probably sinusitis. Now, as an orthopaedic surgeon, this may not have been my field, but as a grandfather with eight grandchildren at the time I told him I knew that snot is usually green or yellow. This stuff was as clear as Evian water. I came home and went to bed. That night I developed the king of all headaches. The pain was so bad that I rolled up in a ball with all the lights off. Freda knew something was badly wrong – and she was right.

I went to see a neurosurgeon and told him about the clear fluid. He wanted me to repeat the trick so I asked him for a glass. Once again it came flowing out of me. I could see the grave look of concern on his face. He took me by the hand and led me straight down the corridor for a scan. The results confirmed his fears. He told me I had a fracture across the base of my skull, all the way from the middle ear to my sphenoidal sinus. He said the dura mater – part of the meninges membrane around the brain – had been holding up for years but had finally given way and spinal fluid was leaking into the sphenoidal sinus and out of the nose. I had the early stages of meningism, a serious condition that causes blinding headaches and can lead to meningitis if it becomes infected. It was the result of concussion suffered in the accident. I'd been fine for nearly twenty-five years and never even had a headache. Then as soon as I retired it suddenly started causing problems. The neurosurgeon didn't pussyfoot around and told me the situation was both serious and urgent – but I knew that already. He couldn't perform the operation I needed and the only other neurosurgeon in the department that day admitted he hadn't done it for ten years. "You're not coming anywhere near me, then!" I thought.

I came home in a bit of a quandary. At least I now knew what the problem was now, but nobody seemed to have any idea how to deal with it. I took some antibiotics and felt safe for the time being. Soon afterwards I received a phone call out of the blue from a man with a Welsh accent. He introduced himself as Elgan Davies and said he was a Consultant ENT Surgeon in Crewe. He had just returned from a meeting at which someone had shown him my scan and his expert diagnosis was both blunt and chilling.

"If you don't have something done you'll be dead from meningitis within a month," he said.

I arranged for my son to take me across to Cheshire to see him. Elgan explained that my brain was now prolapsing through the defect in the dura. It needed to be put back in and then the dura and skull patched up. He clearly had some experience of the condition. He had just signed off an airline pilot who sustained the same injury in a bizarre accident in Iceland. His was stuck out there for a few days while the twin-engined passenger jet he flew was being serviced and had ended up doing the sort of thing bored airline pilots do to pass the time. He wanted to take photographs of his co-pilot messing about in a little Cessna aircraft and in order to get the best picture, he stood on the end of the runway as his mate flew straight at him. Unfortunately, the co-pilot didn't quite time it right and he was struck by the wheel of the plane as it passed, fracturing his skull. Elgan explained that the pilot underwent the operation, rested for three months and was fully healed and able to fly again. It was an encouraging story – but I was still worried sick. If he'd said I had a broken hip or knee I'd have known exactly what to expect, but the thought of someone poking around with my brain didn't excite me at all. Then there were all the possible complications he warned me about. He said there was a danger he could damage my optic nerve, leaving me blind in one eye. Another risk was that I could have fits. But despite those all too real risks, I was reassured by the calm and confidence Elgan exuded. He told me the only time he'd ever felt nervous about the operation I was about to undergo was once when he had to stand by and watch a trainee do it.

I was booked in for surgery the following week and the operation was horrible. Elgan went in through my nose and into the side of my head, found the hole and pushed the prolapsed tissue back up into place. He then inserted some cartilage – part of the septum out of my nose – to bridge the gap. He also used some bone and performed a myofascial temporalis muscle graft from the side of my head to cover everything over and finally, he patched me up again. I woke up in intensive care and looked towards the wall. "At least I can still see the clock," I thought. Next, I raised my hands and wiggled my fingers to make sure they were still working. Everything seemed as it should be. I breathed a tremendous sigh of relief. When I emerged from intensive care I had a catheter in my brain, taped all the way down my back and leading to a bottle of yellow liquid hanging beside my bed. Elgan explained that it was to monitor my spinal fluid.

"Everything went as planned," he said. "We've just got to see if it works now."

That sobering comment made me realise that I was far from out of the woods yet. I was in hospital for eight days. By day six my spinal pressure had normalised sufficiently for the catheter to be removed. But that meant stripping off the full sheet of three-inch Elastoplast that was taping it to my back. It didn't help that I'm like a gorilla, covered all over with hair. The anaesthetist didn't pull any punches.

"This is going to hurt you more than you've ever been hurt before," he said, promising to get it over with quickly.

He was true to his word. It was excruciating. I thought I had earned a Master's degree in pain with the almighty headaches I'd been suffering, but this was sheer agony.

When the time came for me to be discharged, Elgan arranged to see me again in a few weeks and issued instructions to call him if there were any problems. He ordered me to take it easy and to sit up constantly for three months, even when I went to bed. It was a hugely frustrating time for me. I couldn't fly so there would be no holidays as I recuperated. I wasn't allowed to go to the gym and I couldn't drive either, which was infuriating, as I'd just taken delivery of a brand new Land Rover. Three months later I returned to Crewe to get Elgan's verdict on the outcome of his handiwork. I was given the news I was hoping for. After a quick scan, he told me I was cured.

After six weeks he said I could drive again and on the last day of the third month I was back in the gym. I was a bit wary about lying down and straining, as there was a risk I could blow the patch in my brain. Thankfully I've never had any trouble since. I didn't have any fits and there was no damage to my vision. There's always been a joke within the medical profession that orthopaedic surgeons don't have any brains because much of our work is all about brawn as we go at it with our hammers and saws. But as Elgan discharged me from his care he handed me a photograph.

"It's not true what they say about you lot," he said. I was mystified.

"What is it?" I asked.

"It's a picture of your brain," he told me.

While he had the scope up there he decided to take a snap and give it to me. He showed me the tissue that was coming down and explained how he'd been able to push it back.

"What's that white area?" I asked.

"It's your optic nerve," he said.

"And that red one?"

"Your internal carotid artery."

"How far were you away from them?"

"About a millimetre," he smiled.

What a remarkable man! Now one hundred per cent well again, I was able to relax and start spending some quality time with my wife and family. Freda had virtually brought the kids up on her own while I spent every hour God sent at the hospital for forty years. It would have been a cruel twist of fate if she'd lost me on an operating theatre table before we'd had a chance to enjoy our retirement together. Not that she ever resented me being away from home. She felt it was her role to support me, so I could get on with doing what I did best. And I enjoyed every minute of my life behind the mask…

2

War Baby

I was born in Redcar's old Kirkleatham Hospital, which was being used as a temporary maternity unit during the war. My kids always pull my leg and ask, "Which war was that then, Dad?" Well, it was January 21st 1941, the day British and Australian troops recaptured the Libyan town of Tobruk from the Italians in Operation Compass during World War II. I was an only child. Mam told me I had a brother who died when he was very young, probably just after he was born, and was buried in Oxbridge Cemetery in Stockton. Sadly, I've been unable to trace his grave.

Dad's family hailed from East Lothian in the Scottish Borders and came down to the North East because of a shortage of employment in agriculture. His father's first wife died at the age of fifty-two and Dad had two stepbrothers and a step-sister from that marriage before my grandfather married my grandmother. His cousins were all Durham miners and when I was a small child of six or seven we occasionally went up to Easington and Horden on Sunday afternoons for tea. Children were to be seen and not heard up there. We sat in a room with dark curtains, big velvet antimacassar coverings on the furniture and huge aspidistras in the corner. The lads coming in from the pit after their shift washed in a tin bath in the kitchen. Stan Anderson, the only man to have captained all three big North East football teams, Newcastle, Middlesbrough and Sunderland, is a distant relation from that side of the family and I met him when I was very small. While that branch of the Anderson clan came down to Durham and Northumberland, Dad's branch settled in Stockton, where he was born. Grandfather's second wife was Hannah, from the Egton Bridge area, out near Whitby. In her earlier years she was the housekeeper for one of the Catholic parishes in Hull. Grandfather got a job as a locomotive driver in the steelworks and they had two children together, my dad, Thomas William, and his sister, Annie.

Mam was born in Bishop Auckland and was christened Annie Rosina Archer. My grandfather on her side was a railway signalman who lost a leg when he was struck by lightning while he was walking along the track one night. Mam was one of six children. She had four brothers and one sister, Cissy, who died of pneumonia in her twenties. Three of her brothers, Freddy, Les and Billy, followed their dad into the railways while the other one, Tommy, worked for the gas board. Tommy was also the only one of the sons who married and the others stayed with my Gran, Amy, till she died. The family later moved from Port Clarence to Middlesbrough.

Dad worked in Bowesfield Steel Works, which was where Halfords is now, just as you enter Stockton. Mam was a nursing assistant before going into domestic service just off Cambridge Road, very close to where we live now. She once pointed across the road from my house and told me, "Your dad used to stand on that corner waiting to pick me up when I finished work."

Dad was forty when I was born. He was too old to be called up to the services and his job in the steelworks was a reserved occupation anyway. When the steelworks reduced their output he joined the fire service in Redcar.

We lived in a cul-de-sac called Victoria Avenue just near the racecourse. Although I was only there for the first five years of my life, I remember it very well. Our lovely little back garden with its Anderson Shelter always fascinated me. I must have been very young but I remember it being built. We had a black spaniel-type dog called Gyp and it broke my heart when he fell off the railway bridge over Borough Road and was killed.

There were troops billeted around us, staying in houses that had room for them. They were always friendly with the local kids and used to make us toys. One soldier carved me a plane out of a solid piece of wood. I loved it and kept it for years.

Our bedroom window faced south-west. I know that because one night when I was only two or three, Mam held me at the window and shouted for Dad.

"Come and see this," she said. "It's a Doodlebug." That was the nickname British people gave to the dreaded V-1 flying bombs. Thousands of them were launched towards south-east England from German bases on the French and Dutch coasts. The sight was so vivid that I can picture its *do-do-do-do-do* trail right across the sky. I recalled the story many years later and was told I must be mistaken because the V-1s didn't come this far north. Because they had a limited fuse they were usually sent over to terrorise London. But at that stage of the war, when the RAF were destroying their land bases, the Luftwaffe's "Blitz Wing" began carrying them over the North Sea to Hull on modified Heinkel He 111s, pointing them towards the North East and then releasing them. One landed somewhere just north of Darlington. The one we saw was travelling from south-east to solar north-west. Another time Dad took me to see a single-seater fighter plane that had crashed on Redcar beach. I sat high up on his shoulders and was able to touch the rudder. It's little wonder I was fascinated by planes from such an early age.

I started school at Redcar Lane Primary School, walking along Victoria Avenue and crossing the railway line to get there. The boys would all hang onto the gates and swing open with them when the man pulled the lever. It was pretty safe to be out and I played in the street with some of the kids who lived nearby. I'd walk from our house to the sweet shop and tobacconist on the corner of Borough Road. One particularly bad winter a narrow path was cleared along Redcar Lane and the snow at either side was stacked up higher than me. We had to walk through this snow tunnel to get to the sweetshop. There was an old-fashioned cigarette machine at the side of the road, selling Players and Capstans, but when the back came off I decided to have a fiddle about inside. The wires were bare and I got a nasty electric shock, scaring the life out of me. I've been terrified of cigarette machines ever since.

Once peace returned Dad left the fire station and looked for a job with ICI. The sprawling Wilton site near Redcar opened in 1946 to help meet the huge demand for the materials needed to rebuild the country after the war. But instead of getting a job here on our doorstep, he was offered one at the other big ICI complex on Teesside, at Billingham. That meant the family had to up sticks and move from Redcar to Middlesbrough. We lived in Park Lane at first, right opposite Nazareth House children's home, which fascinated us as little lads. My friends and I would look over the wall and see all the girls doing the washing and laundry, or if I was in one of my pal's houses we could see them playing in the garden down the side of the building. We wondered why they were all in there and not at home with their families. Later we bought a house in nearby Abingdon Road. We didn't have a car but I got around on a bike.

Dad was a Catholic and Mam converted to Catholicism to marry him, which you had to in those days. I can still remember my first day at St Joseph's – it's always a bit frightening, moving to a new school. My teacher was Mrs O'Rourke and my classroom is still there on the corner looking out onto Marton Road. I did pretty well at school. In the summer of 1949, when I ended my year in junior one, Sister Monica wrote in my report: "Works steadily, makes fairly good progress." In my Christmas 1949 report from junior two, the teacher wrote: "A keen, intelligent, hard-working boy. Position in class – second. Works well and always does his best. Conduct: Very good." But by the end of that school year I was starting to show my potential. I'll never forget seeing the words: "Position in class – first." There was another boy who always came first. His parents were both teachers, whereas I came from staunchly working-class stock. He suddenly found himself in second place for the first time and he literally fell to the floor when he heard the news. I thought he'd had a fit at first. I suppose he had, but only a hissy fit! Normal service was soon restored, however, and in the last report before I left St Joseph's I'd fallen back to third place.

I enjoyed school. I was well behaved and probably a little bit frightened because the nuns weren't averse to beating you if you stepped out of line – and sometimes even if you didn't. We were whacked regularly. That was the way it was in those days. It didn't do you any harm. I got a few thrashings, usually because my mates got me into mischief. Once we went over the road to one of the houses opposite where a man had an aviary full of budgies. We didn't think that was right. "Why should you keep them in a cage?" we said. So we let a couple of them go. We got thrashed for that – and I mean thrashed!

Another time, I was passing a note to a girl in my class. It said "I love you", but my first attempt at romance ended in tears when someone intercepted it and Sister Baptiste beat me.

My daily walk to school took me past an old sweet shop called Spencer's, opposite the end of Park Lane, near the garage that's still there now. Mr Spencer was a tall, cadaverous man. He looked like an undertaker and always had a dewdrop hanging off the end of his nose. Not that it bothered us kids or put us off buying his wares. Mam gave me ration coupons to hand over because you couldn't buy sweets otherwise. I'd ask for my two ounces of mint humbugs and he'd pour them out of the big jar, into the scales and then into a paper bag, skilfully flipping it over to seal the corners with two little twists. There were always cars parked in the gap where you could turn right out of Park Lane towards Albert Park gates. One day, on our way home from school, the cars were all covered with dust and we decided to write something on them. For some reason I wrote "shit". Unfortunately for me, Miss Hardie was coming past on her bike. We got beaten for that as well.

We were always in and out of Albert Park. There were some roadworks just outside the gates one night and in those days they lit candles and put them in red lamps to warn people about the hole. We watched from Clairville Common as the workmen lit his lamps around the hole. Then, as soon as he'd gone, we ran over and blew them all out. The next thing I knew, a huge hand grabbed my collar from behind me. It was a policeman.

"Got yer!" he said.

The rest of the lads ran away, but he managed to get hold of two of us and gave us a clip round the ear.

"This is a very serious matter," he said sternly. "I'll be coming round your house tonight to see your parents."

I lay awake all night worrying, with my head under the covers. I knew that if he turned up Dad would give me a good hiding as well. That was enough for me to give up my life of crime. It remains the only interaction I've had with the police throughout my life, except for the odd speeding ticket.

St Joe's was a good school and had a real cross-section of society, from the lowest of the low – and I was down in that group – to kids from better families, the sons of doctors and teachers who lived further up Marton Road. It was my first experience of being thrown into the deep end and mixing with a different social class. That was something I was going to have to get used to.

3

The College

One day in June 1952 an official-looking letter dropped onto the doormat at our house in Abingdon Road. Mam opened it up and read it out as Dad and I listened attentively.

"I'm pleased to hear that your son's been awarded a scholarship," it said, welcoming me to St Mary's College. I'd passed the eleven-plus examination that everyone sat at the end of primary school, earning me a place at the grammar school. The college was on The Avenue in Linthorpe, where St Edward's School is now. A couple of my mates from St Joe's went with me but I also made a whole new set of friends from all over the area. I had a nest of pals from South Bank who were a really good clan. One of them was Dimauro, whose father had a shoe repairer's shop on the High Street in South Bank. Dimauro had a beautiful sister called Angela, but he warned us all that he came from Sicily and his family had Mafia connections. He made a menacing throat-cutting gesture with his finger and said that if anyone went near Angela, we were for it – and consequently, nobody did!

Then there was Georgie Williams and Mike Byrne, who lived in Cod Street. Every Friday night I'd pay a couple of pennies to get the trolley bus from the corner of Borough Road and Linthorpe Road and go to South Bank to see Mike. His mam was a character. We did what lads did, smoked illicit cigarettes and then had a drop of beer as we got a bit older. We'd walk around eyeing the girls up and go to the pictures together. They were a good gang of lads and we were very close.

Lads came to the college from further afield, including places such as Lealholm, out on the Whitby Road. Thomas Hodgkinson used to stand on a junction on the Moor Road in the middle of winter, surrounded by snow and waiting for the bus to bring him to college. He was a nice lad but a typical farm boy and we all got a bit of a laugh out of him.

Discipline was strong and there were yet more beatings if you did anything wrong. The physics teacher, Harry Kelly, had one of those big, triangular set squares teachers drew straight lines on the board with. He'd rap it on the desk and if you hadn't done your homework or you got something wrong he'd launch it across the room at you. If your misdemeanour was something worse you'd have to bend over and get a whack in front of the whole class. Father Frank Byrne – who was known as Basher Byrne – was a Marist priest who taught French and was also the discipline master. Every morning when we trooped in for school he would stand brandishing a golf club at the head of the column of boys as it split into two. Anybody who was out of line got a whack with the club. He'd regularly rap the back of your knuckles with a ruler during French lessons.

"Final-consonants-in-French-are-not-pronounced-are-they?" he'd say in a rhythmic, singsong voice.

"No, Father," we'd reply.

"Well-do-not-pronounce-them-then..."

I was never sent to the headmaster's office to be caned, but the masters knocked us about and Harry Kelly wasn't the only one who would throw things at us. The blackboard rubber occasionally came flying through a hole in the partition wall, which we always thought was great fun, as long as you weren't the one it hit.

The war had an enormous impact on all of us who grew up at that time and many of the games we played had a military theme. When we went to the cinema we either watched cowboy films starring Alan Ladd and John Wayne or war films. There were lots of second-hand army stores, selling off all the surplus equipment left over when millions of servicemen were demobbed. One of them was Over The Border, what we called the area of town past the railway station and home to the old St Mary's Cathedral that burned down many years later. You could get your hands on virtually anything in this shop. My pal Bobby Waters and I bought an old set of wartime field phones and rigged them up across the back alley, trailing the wires the fifty yards from our house to his in Waterloo Road. Bobby wasn't a Catholic and went to the High School when I went to St Mary's, but we stayed close. His dad was in the Royal Navy Munitions and Armaments department during the war and enthralled us with stories and tales. Bobby was bright and very good at chemistry and we used to make explosives together. We learned to make exploding potassium iodide that dried into crystals. Then we'd put in on the pavement and frighten the life out of people when it went "Bang!" as they passed. Another time we took the extension pipe from Mam's Hoover and fired rockets out of the tube like a bazooka all the way up the back alley.

When I was fourteen I joined the Air Cadets. It was the natural thing to do for a kid who was as mad about planes as I was, and I loved the excitement. Middlesbrough 1869 squadron was based in a little hut at the top of Clairville Road and Marton Road. It was quite disciplined and we learnt basic services drill and paraded outside the hut. We also went to camps at RAF Syerston, near Nottingham, where I had my first experience of flying in an old training aircraft. They sometimes took us from the Thornaby Aerodrome to Whitby and then up the coast in an old fashioned Anson aircraft, which looked like a Second World War Dakota. I spent hours at Thornaby. I was fascinated by warplanes in particular at a time when the early jets such as the de Havilland Vampire and the Gloster Meteor were coming in. Planes went out on target practice over the North Sea and I'd lie at the end of the runway, waiting for them to return. Unfortunately, one would occasionally hit the top of the Eston Hills in bad weather as it came back. All the Catholic schoolchildren in Middlesbrough took part in the Corpus Christi Procession, which started at the cathedral on a Sunday afternoon every May or June. One year as we walked, Georgie Williamson told me a plane had gone down on the Eston Hills. The second the procession was over we were off as fast as our feet could carry us. When we arrived we collected up whatever bits of the plane that we could. My bedroom was crammed full of crashed aircraft parts. Another time one of my South Bank pals was playing on a slag tip when he came across the site where a plane was brought down by *ack ack* anti-aircraft fire during the war. There was an air raid on the railway station and the air-gunner caught one as it headed back home. My mate found a German pistol, which he gave to me. The handle had burnt off in the fire so we made a new one from wood. The mechanism was charred and had seized up, but we eventually got it working. There was no ammunition, that had exploded in the heat, so Bobby and I tried to melt down my lead soldiers in my shed in Abingdon Road to make some bullets. We took a tobacco tin lid and put some sand in, making an impression for a bullet. But the sand was damp and exploded as soon as the molten lead hit it. Dad heard us shouting and came running down to see what had happened. I got a good hiding for that. But he didn't take the gun off me. Sadly, Mam threw all my aircraft parts and memorabilia out when I went to university.

Next door to us in Abingdon Road were the Allan family, who had three children. Their dad, Bert, had been in the RAF during the war, and because I was into planes in a big way he gave me a pile of the recognition charts pilots used to use to identify the Messerschmitts and Heinkels. I had them all over the walls in my room and got my hands on as many aircraft recognition books as I could.

My first headmaster at St Mary's, Father Philip Symes, was a very nice, tall man who looked like the actor Geoff Chandler with his thick, white hair. His successor, Cyril G Trueman, was a well-educated arty-type, who was into elocution and wanted us all to speak properly. He was determined to rid us of the glottal stop that's such a part of the Middlesbrough accent. It drove us mad. But he also put on plays and I got involved in one somehow. I played Richard, with Jane Taylor opposite me, in Christopher Fry's *The Lady's Not For Burning*, a romantic comedy set in the Middle Ages. I've still got the ticket and programme, signed by the cast. The ticket was two and six and the programme was sixpence, with the profits going "To aid the World Refugee Fund".

I was chosen to be the head boy in my final year at St Mary's. My main achievement during my tenure was getting permission for sixth form boys to have a cigarette – for my sins! I remember going to see the headmaster with our request. Smoking seemed terribly sophisticated in those days.

I worked hard during my school years and continued to do so through college, but I don't know where my work ethic came from. I can't honestly say any of my forebears were particularly hard-working. Dad dismayed me a little bit with his attitude to work. When he was at the ICI I'd be the one who had to ring up to tell them when he was having a "sickie". I was only a kid of ten or twelve and I'd have to say, "Dad's got a cold and he won't be in tonight." I used to think, "How terrible, not going to work just because you've got a cold!" You don't miss work because you've got a bit of a sniffle. I've had that ethos all my life, I've been totally focused on my work. Dad was offered a foreman's job but wouldn't take it. That was something I could never understand during my childhood.

But Dad had a great head for figures and taught me about maths. He would also quote the odd verse from poems he'd learned at school. One of my grandsons, Ollie, was doing a project on the Romans and was told to study *Horatius At The Bridge*. I immediately remembered Dad reeling off one of the epic work's seventy stanzas. The poem was written in 1842 by the Victorian poet Thomas Babington Macaulay and recalls heroic events from Roman history. Horatius the centurion was posted at the gate along with two guards when the Etruscan army arrived to attack Rome. These three soldiers were all that stood between the great city and this mighty army. Horatius told the townspeople to cut the bridge down and they duly hacked away at it. Just as it started to give way, he turned to his two mates, Lartius and Herminius, and said, "You get back, lads." Then the bridge collapsed and he threw himself into the Tiber. Somehow he survived and they pulled him out at the other side. I never forgot it and was amazed when Ollie told me he was studying that same poem. "I'm your man!" I said. Then I thought of Dad and quoted him…

Then out spake brave Horatius,
  The Captain of the gate:
  "To every man upon this earth

THE MAN BEHIND THE MASK

Death cometh soon or late.
And how can man die better
Than facing fearful odds
For the ashes of his fathers
And the temples of his gods"

Bless him. He was a good dad.

4

The Back Story

The big dance at Constantine Technical College every Saturday night was the place for us teenagers to be seen. It was not far from my house, at what's now one of the Teesside University buildings on Borough Road. One night I lifted up a girl I was dancing with and swung her over my head, as was the fashion at that time. But just as I did so an excruciating pain shot down my back. I could hardly move. My dancing partner kindly helped me home and Mam called out the doctor. He didn't like the look of it and asked for a home visit from the consultant Matt Leitch, who would later be my boss. When he examined me he shared the GP's concern.

"I'm not happy about this," he said. "We'll get you into the hospital for a proper investigation."

I was fifteen, too old for a children's ward, so I was sent instead to Middlesbrough General Hospital's ward nine, which was the men's trauma ward. I was the youngest in there by some way and was surrounded by grown men lying on their backs with their legs up in traction after car and motorcycle crashes and other unfortunate accidents. But I was soon at home there and enjoyed the chatter with the blokes. The doctors ordered x-rays and noticed some unusual changes in the vertebrae. Tests revealed I had a raised inflammatory marker in my blood. In those days the big fear with vertebrae problems was tuberculosis, a serious infectious disease that was still a major problem at that time. I was splayed out like a gingerbread man on a spinal frame and I didn't move for nearly a year. It turned out I had Scheuermann's disease, named after the man who discovered it. In tuberculosis, the infection gets in between the vertebrae and the discs in your back and erodes the bone, causing the disc to bulge. Scheuermann's disease has similar symptoms and often occurs in the early teenage years. The bones seem slightly soft and the discs become herniated, resulting in backache, as you would get with TB. It was difficult to distinguish between the two and they treated it as TB until proved otherwise. A child with Scheuermann's today would have a week's bed rest and then be back on his feet again. I went into hospital in January and it was almost Christmas by the time I came back home.

After nine weeks in the General, I was transferred to the Friarage at Northallerton. The Evening Gazette printed a picture of me as a chubby teenager lying in my frame and being pulled around an RAF fair they held in the hospital grounds. Being in hospital for so long played havoc with my education. It was my O level year and I was able to do Maths, French, English, Latin and Geography, passing them all, but I couldn't study any of the scientific subjects, such as physics and chemistry. A vicar's wife from Northallerton came in to teach me French and Latin. I was lying in my frame while we were going through the French oral exam when I got a terrible urge to pee. I called the nurse and she brought me one of those clear glass bottles. But I felt an agonising pain and when I looked down the bottle was full of blood. When you lie still for months on end, calcium crumbles away from your bones into your blood and collects in your kidneys. It had caused a renal stone, which was the most painful thing I've ever had in my life.

It was 1957, the year of the Asian flu pandemic. Nobody had it in Northallerton at that time but my mates brought it with them when they came through from Middlesbrough to visit me. I was the first person in Northallerton to get it and I became quite ill. They put me on antibiotics but discovered I was allergic to penicillin, so I had to have adrenaline injections instead.

It was also the year the Russians launched the first artificial Earth satellite, Sputnik 1, and then Sputnik 2, which saw the first animal in space, Laika the dog. It was an exciting time and breaking speed records was all the rage, with men planning to fly at a thousand miles an hour. I had a book from America about Chuck Yeager, the first pilot confirmed to have exceeded the speed of sound in level flight. He flew the Bell X-1 experimental aircraft, which was like a rocket. They took it up in a B-29 Superfortress and drop launched it from the bomb bay. Yeager zoomed off and reached the speed of Mach 1.06. He also did high-speed tests on the ground as he tried to learn about the effects of high speeds on aircrew. Strapped into a sled, he zipped along at 700 miles an hour before coming to rest in a water bath. When he got out his face was bruised because of the forces of the deceleration. I was absolutely fascinated by these developments. All the way through school I'd always wanted to join the RAF and become a pilot. I'd even filled in an application for an officer cadetship at RAF Cranwell, although I was worried I wouldn't be able to fly because I was wearing glasses by then. At the same time as reading thrilling reports about space exploration and high-speed flight, I was also seeing dashing surgeons including Matt Leitch, Gilbert Parker and Bruno Isserlin treating all these poor children who had crippling illnesses or had suffered terrible accidents. Many of the children were able to get up and walk again afterwards. "That's not a bad job," I thought. By the time I came out of hospital, I'd changed my mind about becoming a pilot. I wanted to be a doctor instead. When I broke the news to Mam and Dad they were very supportive, although they were also absolutely gobsmacked. Dad's idea of elevation in life was becoming a white-collar worker such as a draughtsman in the offices at ICI. That was the job to have in his eyes but it had no appeal for me. I went back to the college and told them I needed the sciences to get into medical school. That meant an extra year studying for O levels in Chemistry and Physics, before moving up to the sixth form and applying for a place at medical school. Father Symes came to see me in hospital and when I told him I'd changed my mind about my future career and wanted to do medicine, he gave me tremendous encouragement.

I only applied to one university. I'd read lots of books about the history of medicine and became very interested in anaesthetics. I was fascinated by accounts of the first operations under anaesthetic when Robert Lister gave people chloroform, including Queen Victoria when she had a baby. They had to chop people's legs off in less than fifty seconds because that's how long the anaesthetic lasted. I was very impressed by that. The first operation under anaesthetic was carried out at University College London, so when the time came to apply that was the only place for me. I'd hardly ever been out of Middlesbrough before, apart from my annual holiday at the seaside. Every summer during my primary school days I stayed with my dad's sister, Annie, and her husband, Joe Segriff, at Heysham, near Morecambe. Joe was a former soldier who was stationed in Palestine during the war. They couldn't have children so they adopted a little girl, Veronica. She was about three years older than me but we were really good mates and I'd stay with them for the whole six weeks. They lived by the seaside and I was always in the sea, exploring among the rock pools or climbing the cliffs. I enjoyed going there and loved the whole area. Our two families went to the Isle of Man once or twice, Joe and Annie, Mam and Dad and Veronica and me. But most years I went to Heysham, spending hours travelling across the Dales to Morecambe on a rattly old train, with my head out of the window so that my face was black with smoke by the time I arrived.

I was given an interview and travelled down to London for my interview by train and staying the night at the YMCA on Tottenham Court Road. I was absolutely captivated by the city. A friend from the sixth form, a Polish lad called Tad Pilicek, had started at King's College the year before and promised to show me around London. I believe we were the first two St Mary's College boys to study medicine. Tad took me to Soho, which in those days really was a den of iniquity, believe me. For a lad from the provinces to see the girls standing around was something of an eye-opener, to say the least. It was all new to me but not to Tad, who impressed me with his worldliness and sophistication as he got into some witty exchanges with the girls.

The interview process involved a lengthy and rigorous assessment by a large panel, including the Dean of the Medical School and a couple of doctors. I was pretty knowledgeable about UCH, having read so much about it. I told them I was interested in anaesthetics and they could tell I was well-versed in what was going on in the field. They offered me a place on the spot. I had

THE BACK STORY

to pass my A levels but they didn't ask for certain grades, as they do now. I wasn't particularly keen on sport when I was younger but lots of kids got into the London medical schools in those days because they were good at rugby. There was a terrific rivalry between the schools such as St Thomas, Guys and Bart's. Also, if your father had studied there you were pretty much guaranteed a place. So it was quite a breakthrough for me to get in, coming from a solidly working-class background. I was mixing with people from completely different social strata to anything I'd experienced before. Their parents were all professional people and there were probably only three or four of us from state schools out of seventy students in the year. The rest were all privately educated and their fathers were businessmen, doctors and lawyers. I was completely overawed and felt out of place when I first arrived. I thought, I can't tell them all about my school, or my house, or what we'd done, in the way all this lot do. But those feelings soon passed and I made some good friends and got on well with everybody.

We spent the first eighteen months in the dissecting rooms and physiology and chemistry labs and listening to lectures. After that, we did our clinical work and went into the hospital. Each of us joined a "firm" of maybe six which was attached to a consultant. UCH was a big old Victorian hospital, with tiled walls and huge staircases. We'd wait together at nine o'clock in the morning for our boss to pull up in his Bentley. The consultant in my firm was a well-established cardiovascular physician, who looked after the heart and circulation. He would walk in and hand his briefcase to whichever poor student had been pushed to the front. Then he'd gallop up the stairs and we all had to run after him, including the poor lad carrying his case.

"Gentleman," he declared one day. "If you want to live a long time, make sure you get out of breath at least once every day."

"Does that include sex as well?" came a voice from some joker at the back of the group.

After eighteen months there was an intake of about fifty students from Oxford and Cambridge, so the class became about 120. There were only six girls in that whole group. It's totally changed now and around eighty per cent of medical students are girls, which is a good thing because medicine is a great job for women.

In my second year, I was elected secretary of the University Medical Society. "I'm not doing badly in this new world," I thought.

We did a fair bit of drinking, as you do. I somehow got myself co-opted into the UCH hockey team, playing in goal, and we went to the annual hockey festival in Jersey. Thousands of students from all over the country converged there and it was a great place to buy duty-free booze and fags to bring back home. One of my pals, Alan Early, whose father was the headmaster of Kingston Grammar in Hull, was a brilliant musician who could play just any instrument he picked up. We decided to form a folk group together. I hadn't played any musical instruments but I had a good singing voice and learned basic chords on a folk guitar. We adopted another guy called Ricky Cawood, only because he'd been left a couple of thousand pounds by his aunt and could afford to buy a fantastic recording set-up. We had a great time. We recorded our songs down in the basement of the medical school and then got bookings to play all over the place. It was the days of the folk revival and everyone was listening to people like Bob Dylan, the Everly Brothers and Peter, Paul and Mary. We played at parties for a few quid a time, put on a show at the nurses' home and played all night on a boat on Regent's Canal. We even sent a disc off to a record company and got a reply back from them. "It's not bad," it said. "But don't give up the day job!" I've still got all my songbooks and two or three guitars, although I can't play anymore because of arthritis in my fingers.

The Post Office Tower was being built and when I eventually got into the hostel in Gower Street my room overlooked the site. I watched it going up slowly over the years I was studying. When it was completed it was Britain's tallest building and my sister-in-law took us for dinner in the restaurant at the top to celebrate my qualification.

It was a wonderful time in my life and I enjoyed every minute. Right at the end, in my final internal exams, I got an honour in surgery known as *Proxime Accessit*. It means "Almost made it" – I'd come second in the whole year.

As we approached graduation, with our final exams looming, a poster went up on the noticeboard saying the RAF were desperate for doctors. With my lifelong love of planes, it was a hugely attractive opportunity. I wasn't thinking of committing myself for life, but a short service commission was very appealing. I decided to go for it.

5

Falling for Freda

I first set eyes on the love of my life at Constantine College. To get into medical school at that time you needed A levels in Botany, Zoology, Latin, Physics and Chemistry. Botany was so you understood about plants from a pharmacological point of view, Zoology was learning about living species and the Latin was because that was the language all the scripts were written in. As a Catholic that wasn't a problem for me. We went to Mass every week and the service was still in Latin in those days. In any case, everybody learned Latin up to O level at school. But they didn't teach Botany or Zoology at St Mary's College, so they arranged for me to go to Constantine College one or two afternoons a week to study them. Freda also wanted to do a degree that required those subjects and she was sent to Constantine from the Convent, where Catholic girls who passed the scholarship went. Our first date is forever etched on my mind. It was on March 9th 1959 and we went to see *The Nun's Story*, with Audrey Hepburn and Peter Finch, at the Odeon.

Freda was born in July 1940, just a few months before me. Although she went to the same primary school as me, I didn't know her then because she was a school year older. We always called her Freda but she was actually christened Margaret Elfreda, after a nun her family knew. She lived opposite the old telephone exchange on Marton Road and we would walk down to the Odeon and back together. By coincidence her second name was also Anderson. They were a very religious family and she had four sisters, Betty,

Nancy, Nora and Ena, which was short for Philomena. Her brother Terry was killed in the Mediterranean during the Second World War. Freda was a late arrival. After Terry died, her mother wanted another baby, hoping it would be a boy. Instead, Freda came along. One of her sisters entered a nunnery but later came out again. Another was successful in business, running a second-hand clothes shop called Stothards, in North Ormesby. They were a great bunch of girls and I got on very well with the whole family. People joke about mothers-in-law but I couldn't fault mine. She was an honest old lady of Irish descent and I think she was happy to see her daughter with somebody like me. Freda's father had died at the age of just fifty-three, while she was a teenager, so I never met him. The sisters were very, very close and they all looked after their mother.

Before I could begin my RAF service I had to complete my training. That meant a pre-registration year working in a hospital, six months in surgery and six months in medicine. Freda and I had courted all the way through my studies and I wanted to come back to Middlesbrough to get married, so I did these "house jobs" in the old North Ormesby Hospital.

We were married by Father Fitzgibbon at the old St Mary's Cathedral in Sussex Street, Middlesbrough, on April 2nd 1966. Freda's never forgiven me because I could only get a week off for our honeymoon. We went to Scarborough and stayed at The Grand – and in those days, it really was grand. We returned years later and that grandeur had faded dramatically – everyone was drinking pints of lager and playing bingo. But back then it was a magnificent old-fashioned hotel, with the famous bandleader Max Jaffa and his trio playing while we had our afternoon tea.

Our first home was in hospital accommodation at a house on Westbourne Grove, North Ormesby, just down the road from St Alphonsus Church. From the very start of our marriage I was at work an awful lot of the time. There were two of us looking after sixty patients in two wards at North Ormesby, but my colleague had a medical condition that meant he would often go missing or not turn up for a week at a time. There were operations to carry out during the day and sometimes emergencies in the early hours. Then I'd have to be back again ready when the consultant came in for his ward round at nine o'clock in the morning, to update him on what had happened overnight. We'd go to theatre and do a clinic together and I'd be on call again that night.

I trained under some great old surgeons at North Ormesby, including the chief, Sam Mottershead, Jack Edmondson, Jimmy Oldfield, Alan Tooley and Gordon Fordyce, and then there were the physicians such as Ralph Wilsdon and Clifford Astley. I gained a wealth of surgical experience during my training as I worked with great people like that. The principle was to watch one, do one together and then do one yourself. That was it. And you learnt a lot that way. The other important thing was that your boss was always around somewhere – they never left you completely alone and they were there if you wanted them. I'd finish my routine ward work at North Ormesby and then at seven or eight at night I'd go to Eston Children's Hospital, where there might be six kids waiting to have their appendixes removed. I was once operating there when the theatre doors swung open at midnight. Jimmy Oldfield had called in on his way home from a dinner party.

"Everything all right, John?" he asked, dressed immaculately in his evening suit.

"Fine thank you, Mr Oldfield."

You're not allowed to leave trainees on their own now, you have to stand outside the theatre door. I can honestly remember weeks when I did 168 hours on call – and I hear young lads complaining now! Of course, you do get tired and you have to be careful not to make mistakes. It's true that the work is more technical these days, so there's more scope for things to go wrong. The different branches of medicine have become highly specialised and you can't be a jack-of-all-trades and a master of none. In a way we were jacks-of-all-trades in the past, I suppose. But that really laid down the foundations for the way I continued throughout my working life. People were ill, and illness occurs twenty-four hours a day, seven days a week, so you have to be there and you just got on with it. I turned my hand to whatever was required. Now doctors specialise in one area and wouldn't dream of doing anything else. But it was exciting and I loved it.

I was a newly qualified doctor but also a pilot officer. The RAF paid me a salary as I completed my training so I got a few hundred quid more than the NHS lads, which was a bonus. That meant I was able to buy a second-hand car from Gerry Geraghty, who taught with Freda. It was an Austin 16, a real gangster's car, with running boards, curtains, pop-up headlights and indicators that flicked out at the sides. I paid twenty-five quid for it and it was a brilliant car that just kept on going. One day I was coming back from my sister- in-law's at Billingham and the clutch went. My brother-in-law Rog, who was a TV repairman, came and took us home. Then he went to the Austin shop, at the garage opposite the Coronation Hotel, bought a little shackle costing about ten bob, and put it in himself. We drove the car away again afterwards and it kept on going for many more happy miles. But it was wings, rather than wheels, that would dominate the next few years of my life.

6

Flying High

Once my year's training was up I was the RAF's man. I underwent induction and a three-month officer training course at Cranwell in Lincolnshire, learning how to march and drill. It was n thrilling time to be entering the service. The powerful and futuristic Avro Vulcan strategic bomber carried Britain's first nuclear weapon, the Blue Danube gravity bomb. Together with the Valiant and the Victor, the three aircraft were known as V-Bombers. When we were given a tour of a V-Bomber station, we were told in no uncertain terms, "That's an atom bomb – don't touch it!"

Then the time came for us to receive our postings. They asked what I wanted to do and I told them I had an interest in anaesthetics. But when news of my posting was delivered, it came as a major disappointment. I thought they said I was off to Machrihanish. I knew that was a village on the west coast of Scotland and I wasn't impressed.

"No," they said. "*Muharraq*. It's in Bahrain. On the Persian Gulf."

That sounded rather more interesting. On the downside, it was an unaccompanied year. I couldn't take Freda, which irritated me – especially as she was three months pregnant at this time. Instead, she went home to live with her mother and started her teaching career at St Joseph's, where we both went to school.

RAF Muharraq was a staging post, one of many Britain still had dotted throughout the Middle East, and I was anaesthetist to a newly opened hospital. My boss was the only other doctor on the base, a crusty old Wing Commander who could be a miserable bugger, although he was very nice to me. When he found out Freda was pregnant he encouraged me to bring her out to stay for a few weeks. We were given what were known as "indulgence flights" in the forces, which meant taking advantage of one of the constant transport services leaving RAF Brize Norton in Oxfordshire. Freda managed to get a seat on a Bristol Britannia and all I had to pay was £12 for her meals during the flight. But she was suffering from terrible morning sickness and a fourteen-hour flight on a bumpy old Britannia was the last thing she needed. She was due to arrive in Bahrain on Christmas Eve, but when the plane stopped to refuel in Cyprus the pilot was worried about her condition.

"I think we'll have to offload you and get you to hospital," he said.

But she'd come all that way and was determined to complete her journey, however difficult it was.

"Don't you even think about putting me off this plane!" she told him firmly.

It was great to be reunited with her on Christmas Eve. We spent Christmas Day in blazing sunshine on the Sheikh's Beach, which officers were allowed to use for leisure if we had any time off. It was wonderful. After that we went down every day to sunbathe and enjoy a picnic together. Being able to spend time on the Sheikh's Beach was a great perk, but you had to remember you were guests in another country. I've always said that when you're in someone else's country you respect their rules, whether you agree with them or not. And if you stepped out of line in Bahrain, there was a price to play. Joe, an East African Indian navigator from one of the transport squadrons, was once caught swigging from a bottle of beer on the Sheik's Beach and arrested. The RAF did nothing about it, leaving him to be dealt with by the local authorities.

"Sorry Joe, you've broken the rules," he was told. "You do not drink alcohol here."

He was put in a hole in the ground a little island a few miles off the coast, where he stayed for three days. Hopefully, it taught him a lesson.

When Freda came out the other wives quickly told her she couldn't wear the clothes she'd brought with her. The next afternoon we went straight down to see an Indian tailor at the souk in Manama.

"My wife needs three dresses with full-length sleeves," I told him. They were ready in two hours for a couple of quid.

Inside the base itself we were allowed to drink. Guys regularly went backwards and forwards to Kuwait and brought alcohol back to the Mess. Even when we entertained the Sheik at a social event we could drink alcohol normally, while he would sip orange juice.

The Wing Commander and his wife put us up on the station for a week, then we got a better offer. One of my mates, Flight Lieutenant Pete Day, was a trainer in 208 Fighter Ground Attack Squadron. They flew Hunter FGA.9s and their motto was "Vigilant". Their colours were pale blue and yellow – blue for the sky and yellow for the desert sands, as it was based in the Middle East for most of its long history. They adopted me as their squadron doctor/flight surgeon. There were two trainers attached to the squadron and they would often take me on trips. When Pete had to take his aircraft back to the UK for servicing he invited Freda and me to stay in the little flat-roofed cottage in the village where he and his wife lived.

It was lovely to have her out there with me. I had a little Fiat 500 and we went all over the tiny island together. We did have one scare during her visit. I was on duty at the hospital on the station and she rang me up in a state of sheer panic. There were guns going off outside and people were shouting and banging drums. As it turned out there was no need to be concerned. It was only the locals celebrating *Eid al-Fitr*, the end of Ramadan. Over the next few days we took part in events being held around the town to mark the festival. The celebrations were spectacular, if occasionally a little bit dangerous. Men were dancing and throwing handfuls of black gunpowder into rifles. "If anybody lights a fag round here, the whole lot of us will go up!" I thought.

Our first son, Richard, was born in June 1967. I got a week's leave to come home when he was born at Parkside Maternity Hospital. Even though I'd delivered babies myself, expectant dads were chased away in those days. The Cambridge Hotel had just opened and was quite a posh place. So I went with my childhood friend Bobby Waters, God rest him, to celebrate with a few pints as I waited for my first born to put in an appearance. But before long I was back in Bahrain. The Squadron Commander when I arrived was Tony Chaplin and when he left Jim McVie replaced him. Coincidentally, Jim's son is now an orthopaedic surgeon at James Cook Hospital. Tony and Jim were both big men and I always had a job squeezing into a Hunter cockpit beside Tony. There was also a shortage of large-sized g-suits and you had to wear one, otherwise you'd black out every time they turned the plane. Most of my flights were with Pete, who took me up with him when he went out instructing.

Occasionally, I was asked to assist when someone was taken ill on a ship in the Gulf. One time the captain of a big tanker was sick and I was asked if I'd drop onto the ship by parachute.

"Not on your life," I told them. "If God had meant me to fly I'd have wings!"

So they took me by high-speed RAF launch instead. It was an enormous quarter-of-a-million tonne tanker and I had to climb a hundred feet up a narrow ladder to get on board. It beat being dropped down from a great height though!

The Six-Day War between Israel and several Arab nations took place while I was in Bahrain and I treated several Egyptian pilots who were shot down and had spinal crush fractures. The injuries were as a result of placing cushions on their ejector seats to make them more comfortable. You don't get people doing that in the Royal Air Force. They just put up with the discomfort! But the Egyptian pilots thought it was much better with a cushion on – until they were forced to bale out under attack. An ejector seat is an extremely sensitive piece of equipment in both mechanical and electronic terms. It's assembled using the known force of the rocket and the average weight of the pilot. The cushion is made of a special material that ensures the pilot isn't hurt when he ejects. If you put something else on top of that it completely alters the dynamics and the spine is compressed much more on deployment. If you compress the bones in your lower back you break them, and that's what these guys were doing. Almost the entire Egyptian air force was destroyed during that short conflict that redrew the map of that part of the Middle East.

One of the highlights of my year in the Gulf was receiving an Air Officer's

Commendation for helping to contain a smallpox outbreak. I'd been shipped down to Sharjah, which is now part of the United Arab Emirates, because something had happened to the medical officer there. RAF Sharjah was a staging post for nuclear bombers and came under the direction of RAF Bahrain. At that time they were extending the runway so that Vulcan V-Bombers could come from England, refuel in the Gulf and then fly on as far as the Far East or Russia if they needed to. To carry out the construction work they brought about four thousand Arab workers onto the base every day. But very soon after the work began there was a smallpox epidemic in the local town, Manama. We'd never seen smallpox during my training. A programme of mandatory vaccination had wiped it out in England by the start of the twentieth century. But it was still a major threat to life in many parts of the world. That year alone an estimated fifteen million people contracted this horrific, infectious disease – and two million died. We were bringing four thousand unidentified people onto the base every day to work and when the outbreak was confirmed there was total panic. This was a major RAF base and a staging post for nuclear bombers and we had to prevent an epidemic taking hold. Apart from an old English doctor who had been in the town for many years looking after the local Arab hospital, I was on my own. I immediately put my training into practice. I wasn't long out of medical school and fortunately UCH London had a world-famous School of Tropical Medicine. Having never seen smallpox in England it's quite frightening to be suddenly caught up in the middle of a major outbreak. But I knew that the key to stopping the disease was to isolate known cases and vaccinate everyone who lived close by. It's a process known as "ring vaccination". Vigilance and containment were both crucial. At the camp entrance there were six doorways. I arranged for me, the sergeant and the corporal from sick quarters and three other staff to man the doorways. Every morning we inspected the entire workforce as they arrived. It was vital that nobody with smallpox was allowed in or out of the base.

"Strip them to the waist and take their temperatures," I instructed. "We're looking for spots. If they're clear, let them come in."

We ran out of smallpox vaccine and called for further supplies to be sent out from England urgently. It eventually arrived in the fuel tank of an aircraft, which was usually the method of bringing in booze. When they brought whisky back from Kuwait it was always carried in empty fuel tanks.

The diary of Flight Lieutenant Anderson for March 10th 1967 reads: "Smallpox outbreak. Mass vaccination of all civilians between five o'clock and nine o'clock. Two thousand doses used." I'd then drawn a diagram showing the procedures I'd introduced to screen workers coming through the gates.

They sent a representative from the World Health Organisation in Geneva, who said I was doing everything I should be. Thankfully the measures I took were successful and the disease didn't get onto the base. But I saw lots of smallpox cases and many years later in the 1990s, when terrorists were threatening to send the smallpox virus through the post, they called me into the hospital and asked if I'd be willing to help. I couldn't believe what they were asking me.

"You've got to be joking," I said. "You pay consultants in tropical medicine and you're asking an orthopaedic surgeon?"

But none of them had ever seen smallpox for real. That was just one of the many times my military background stood me in good stead during my long career back in Civvy Street.

7

In the Line of Fire

If you're not frightened when you're rattling through a war zone in an armoured RAF Mini, with flashes and bangs going off all round you, you're not human. That was what I experienced many times when I was sent to what is now Yemen in the Indian Ocean during the Aden Emergency. It was 1967 and a scary time to be there, the height of a fierce insurgency that within months would bring an end to 128 years of British rule. The uprising was in its fourth year but had recently escalated as the Front for the Liberation of Occupied South Yemen tried to force a British withdrawal. It was similar to the situation during Northern Ireland's Troubles. Three flight-sergeants had stopped to fill up their cars as they returned to their quarters after working all day at the RAF base. Terrorists came up and assassinated them at close range, *one-two-three*, just like that. Using the classic assassin's *modus operandi,* two bullets were dispatched through the back of the head and one through the chest.

There were 3,500 British troops stationed in Aden, but their families had been evacuated shortly before I arrived because of the rising security threat. I was sent for because they needed an anaesthetist urgently. I was put in a house in a compound on the base with the senior surgeon, Wing Commander Chris Farrier, and a couple of education officers. The nurses lived in another house across the way. Things were so bad that it wasn't safe to go out at night and we were all told we must learn how to use a weapon.

"Doctors don't shoot," I told them, remembering my Hippocratic Oath.

But this was no ordinary situation. They insisted we had to be capable of protecting our patients if we came under attack. That was the end of the argument and we went down to the range to undergo basic training. I was given a Smith and Wesson .38, but Chris must have expected to be in the thick of the action. He was handed a Thomson submachine gun instead. We blasted away at static targets until we were signed off to carry a sidearm. Once darkness fell, hand grenades and rockets rained in over the fence of the compound. The toilet was down the corridor and one night I was desperate for a pee. But I could hear Chris in his room rattling the slide of his Thomson machine gun and I was terrified to leave my room. You certainly didn't go out of the window because someone outside might take a pot shot at you. So I had to pee in the sink, something I hadn't done since I was a medical student.

The RAF Hospital at Khormaksar Beach received lots of gunshot victims and people with hand grenade injuries. That helped me gain wartime missile-wound experience, which doctors don't get nowadays unless they go to Afghanistan. The main danger for me was getting there at night. We had to go through Sniper Alley, the Ma'alla Strait, where enemy snipers would be lying in wait. We were taken in a little RAF Mini with a roundel on the side, which made a perfect target. As well as the driver there was a guy with an automatic weapon riding shotgun.

The Crater district of Aden was built on the site of an extinct volcano crater. It was abandoned by the British after some soldiers were murdered by mutineering police who were angry that Britain had supposedly supported Israel in the Six-Day War. After that the rebels made their base there. As you approached the town there was constant incoming gunfire from the Crater, which was terrifying. First we'd see a flash but because light travels so much more quickly than sound we didn't hear the bullet coming. By the time you heard a zipping noise through the air it was too late – if it was meant for you, you were dead. We could see flashes all the time and knew each one meant a rifle was going off somewhere, even if it was a couple of miles away. There was a huge sense of relief whenever I arrived safely at the hospital – and a feeling of dread when I knew it was time to go back home again.

The danger of being killed was all too real. Before one officers' mess night the dining room was laid out with a head table for the Commanding Officer and top brass and further tables for everyone else. Mess nights in the forces are great occasions, with everyone dressing smartly in their special mess kit. Thankfully, somebody spotted something suspicious hanging out underneath the edge of a table. A search revealed that the whole place was rigged with plastic explosives and the attack was foiled. Security got really tight after that. The Battle of the Crater began in July 1967. The Argyll and Sutherland Highlanders, led by Lieutenant-Colonel Colin Campbell Mitchell, who became known as "Mad Mitch", went in and emptied the Crater area of all the baddies. Not long after that Britain withdrew from Aden.

After a month in Aden I returned to Bahrain. Life was generally much quieter there but I still had the odd heart-stopping moment. The SAS sometimes brought prisoners they'd picked up in Aden to be treated in our hospital. Once they flew someone in for questioning who had been shot in the neck. I went out in an RAF bus with a reinforced floor to meet the aircraft. The bus was painted in desert colours rather than the usual air force blue. It was about a mile from the end of the runway to the hospital.

"You'd be advised to lie on the floor in case we get attacked, Doc," the RAF Regiment driver told me. We carried the prisoner out of the aircraft, took him back to the hospital and got him prepared for theatre. For what is probably the only time in my life the theatre doors were locked from the outside. It was nighttime and I could see orange sodium lights and the shadows of men walking past the frosted theatre windows. It was only then that I realised they had armed guards positioned around the theatre to protect this suspect who they didn't want to lose. Once he was ready for surgery I fished the bullet out and sewed him up again. He didn't have any long-term damage so they could then take him off for interrogation.

The SAS were a tough bunch. When they dressed as Arabs their disguises were so good that our own men would sometimes fire at them, so we got the odd injured Special Forces man in. They were the only people who wouldn't talk when you put them to sleep. We used pentothal in those days to sedate patients while we put the mask and the tube down them before operating.

Pentothal is sometimes knowns as the "truth drug" because people will tell you anything once they're under its influence. But the SAS had been trained to resist saying anything. Once they got pentothal in them they sat bolt upright and gave you their name and number. That was it. You'd get no more information out of them.

I was also sent was Muscat, the capital of Oman. I'll never forget the approach as you came in to land there. The pilot had to line up twin peaks in a mountain range and fly in between them. We flew in a big old Blackburn B-101 Beverley heavy transport plane that looked like a bumblebee, with a bulbous body and enormous fins at the back. There was only me sitting in the belly because they were normally used as cargo planes. It was an exhilarating experience as I watched the wing tips narrowly miss the rocky mountain tops as we came in.

Britain was helping to put down the Dhofar Rebellion, which began in 1962 against the Sultanate of Muscat and Oman and was to last fourteen years. The British raised a paramilitary force known as the Trucial Oman Scouts, which had operated in the region in the past, to help suppress the uprising. Services personnel were posted there for a year and were often promoted as an incentive to go. I went out with the Scouts on medical safaris into the desert, part of a strategy to win "hearts and minds". We drove out from the sick quarters in a couple of Land Rovers with an officer from the Trucial Oman Scouts and an Arab driver. We disappeared into the desert following wadis, which are dried up river beds, while the drivers navigated by the stars. It was a remarkable experience. We visited Bedouin encampments where we always received a warm welcome and were served coffee and sweetmeats. We'd been taught all the local etiquette and knew to take our shoes off and sit with our feet away from the centre of the table. We found out who was ill and gave them free treatment. There was a lot of tuberculosis about and we examined sufferers and gave them antibiotics. They never came for a follow up in the hospital but it was good for political relations between the British and the local people. The only form of transport for many of the Arabs was by donkey. Believe it or not, donkeys get pneumonia in cold, wet weather, which I was surprised to discover they did get out there in the middle of the desert. The sound of their barking cough would go right through you. If the only form of transport you have is a donkey and it dies, it's a big loss. I was instructed to give them antibiotics for their donkeys.

"I'm not a vet," I complained.

"Come on," the CO insisted. "The other doctors all do it."

I was also flown to Masirah Island, about fifteen miles off the coast of Oman, to treat a tanker captain who had suffered a heart attack. Once I'd got the man stabilised we sat on the veranda outside the officers' mess for a drink. There was half a coconut tree nearby, all splintered and almost falling over. Eventually curiosity got the better of me and I asked what had happened.

"Oh, we were sitting here having a drink one night and the rebels sent a rocket over," I was cooly informed.

The officer pointed to the lights twinkling on the mountain range in the distance. He said that was the fighters. Hunter jets were sent to fly over and try to flush them out of the caves.

The Sultan of Oman and Muscat, Said bin Taimur, was eventually deposed by his son, Qaboos bin Said, in a coup in 1970. Qaboos trained at Sandhurst Military Academy and was very English-orientated and brought in sweeping reforms. The rebellion finally ended in 1976. Although it had failed, Oman had changed forever.

After that first year I came back to the UK and was based at an RAF hospital Cosford, near Wolverhampton, where we were given comfortable, four-bedroom married officer's quarters.

Not long afterwards I received a letter from the air officer in charge of medicine saying they needed a surgeon at RAF Gan, another staging post, in what is now the Maldives. The medical officer's wife was having a baby and needed him home for a while. I didn't want to leave my wife and baby son so soon after coming home and confided in the CEO of the hospital in the bar that night.

"I don't want to go," I told him. "I've just come back from an unaccompanied year in Bahrain and I've been away from my wife for a whole year."

If I was looking for sympathy, I certainly didn't get any.

"If you can't take a joke Anderson, you shouldn't have joined the bloody

RAF," he said bluntly. In the end, they found someone else to go instead. We later got an impressive female commanding officer of the hospital, Group Captain Elspeth Mavor McKechnie, who was something of an amazon and later became an Air Commodore and was awarded the CBE.

At Cosford I started my specialist surgical training and was operating every day. At the same time I was studying for my Fellowship of the Royal College of Surgeons. My old boss at North Ormesby Hospital, Sam Mottershead, once said to me, "Anderson, make sure you come out of the forces with something you didn't go in with."

I thought it was a joke – did he mean the pox or something? He actually meant getting the letters FRCS after my name. After gaining a medical qualification as a doctor you join either the FRCP – the Royal College of Physicians – or the FRCS – the Royal College of Surgeons. It was very wise advice and I completed my training while I was in the RAF. That meant I had a head-start on a lot of blokes my age who didn't have it.

During my time at Cosford I also persuaded my boss that we should make ourselves useful to the local civilian population and I started an injection clinic to treat varicose veins. After around eighteen months I was sent back to Bahrain, where they needed a surgeon for a couple of months. Chris Farrier, my old mate from Aden, was there and I had several other friends among the physicians. I was friendly with the squadron but they had their own medical officer by then. I operated at the hospital every day and also ran clinics. While I was there the Warrant Officer's son got acute appendicitis and became very ill with peritonitis. We had no option but to operate there and then. He did very well and after the boy recovered the Warrant Officer took me into the stores. It was like an Aladdin's Cave, with every surgical tool you could name on display. I remember seeing a brand new Mark 3 Boyle's anaesthetic machine, which was the in thing at the time. It had never been used and still had the clingfilm on. It was worth thousands.

"Doc," he said. "Whatever you want is yours!"

"I can't steal things," I said. He was insistent. He said the British would be leaving the country within a year and everything would be either taken by the Arabs or dumped in the sea. He said he would send whatever I wanted back to Brize Norton, marked for the attention of Flight Lieutenant Anderson. But I couldn't do it. Shortly after that I left and a few months later Bahrain was handed back. A couple of airmen bought two brand new, bomb-proof Land Rovers very cheaply and drove them back over land with their mates when the base closed. But everything I had seen was dumped in the sea. The only thing I did come back with was new golf clubs. When aircraft went to the Far East for servicing the crews were able to buy things cheaply. Someone brought me back a fantastic set of clubs for thirty quid. There was no grass out there, so the Americans used sand and oil to create grey-black greens, which were incredibly fast, like a billiard table. They tried to persuade me to play but it wasn't for me.

My last detachment was to Masirah Island for a couple of weeks. It was yet another staging post, right on the tip of the Gulf, where it meets the Indian Ocean. In those Cold War days it was important that they were all maintained and gave Britain the ability to fly planes to wherever they needed them across the globe. I could fish off the end of the rocks in my spare time and the food was wonderful, an endless supply of beautiful crayfish collected from the rock pools.

I thoroughly enjoyed my RAF career. They were thrilling times for a young Middlesbrough lad just out of medical school. I could have stayed on at the end of my commission. But even though I was still mad about planes, I was even more keen on surgery by then and an exciting new life awaited me.

8

Down to the Bones

When my time in the RAF came to an end I decided that orthopaedics was where my future lay. I had a go at virtually everything in the forces. I opened heads, chests and abdomens. I was sent to areas of the world where I was required to do military surgery after bomb, rocket and hand grenade blasts, as well as treating bullet wounds from rifles and pistols. I also performed a wide variety of general surgery, including cartilage and ligament operations on young men who'd been injured playing sport, as well as treating many members of the local population wherever I was based.

At that time, in the late 1960s and early 1970s, joint replacement was very much in its infancy, but big advances were being made and knee and hip replacements were being introduced throughout the country. I took a keen interest in developments because Dad's sister Annie, in Heysham, had severe rheumatoid arthritis and two grossly deformed knees. Her legs were so stiff that they wouldn't let her on buses because she would trip people up. She struggled to get up out of a chair, although she was a colonel in the St John Ambulance and still managed to go on parade. The way I saw things, joint replacement was the future. People had experimented for years but it was really taking off and I wanted to get involved and take it forward. In those days there was no fixed training programme. You qualified, got the experience, climbed up the ladder, and when they thought you were ready you got a job as a registrar, which is on the bottom rung of the specialist training ladder. Now you do a set four-year training period and then you're a consultant, even though you don't have that much practical experience. In our day it was more like an apprenticeship. I initially decided to go to London because I'd studied there. I applied for a job at the Royal Free Hospital and was given a very rigorous interview, as was the way in those days. But I was turned down and the job went to someone who was already working at the hospital instead. After the interview, Mike Freeman, who was a world expert in the field of knee joints, called me back in for a word.

"I would have given you the job, " he said. "But I'll give you a tip. If you're planning to go back and settle in the North East, I'd look for a job up there if I were you."

It was good advice and Mike and I have remained friends ever since. But despite what he had said, I thought about starting off in Stoke-on-Trent instead. There was an orthopaedic surgeon there called Denys Wainwright, who had done some very interesting hip fracture work and invented the Wainwright spline, which was used in an operation we did for arthritis back in the Stone Age. Freda and I drove down to have a look around but we didn't like the place at all and we came back up to Teesside.

Eventually I got a job as an orthopaedic registrar at Leeds General Infirmary and we set up home in Alwoodley, on the outskirts of the city. By now our family was growing and the money in the NHS wasn't fantastic. To supplement my wages I took on as much extra work as I could, including night shift sessions in the Casualty Department at Bradford Royal. One day I saw a notice on the hospital wall. "Locum wanted, good pay". I rang up and arranged a visit. There I met Dr John Devlin, a large Irish GP who looked after the people who lived in Quarry Hill House, which at that time was Britain's largest social housing complex. As we chatted I noticed a Rolls Royce parked outside the surgery window. Standing beside it was a little old war veteran wearing a beret and an army greatcoat with his medals proudly pinned onto its front. Dr Devlin saw me looking out and the puzzled expression on my face.

"Oh, he's there to stop the little buggers coming along and scratching it," he said. "It's a rough area. The policemen go round in threes here."

I took the job and worked alternate weekends. I'd do the Friday evening surgery if I was off duty and then his Saturday morning surgery and calls. It was an enormous singlehanded practice. John's wife was also a doctor but she no longer worked and they had one teenage daughter. He was a good old-fashioned GP and a wonderful character. When sales reps left him samples he'd take them to the local chemist and exchange them for a pair of Scholl sandals to wear on his holidays or something else that took his fancy. He had a big captain's table with a drawer I could never open until one day when it finally budged. There before my eyes was something of a treasure chest. It was crammed with half-crowns that patients had given for dispensing sick notes. They had built up over the years and must have been worth a fortune!

John gave me a wonderful piece of advice about treating patients that I've never forgotten.

"I'll give you a tip," he said. "Never let the buggers leave the surgery empty-handed. If they come to see the doctor, they expect to go out with something. And this is what I give them – Dr Devlin's Special White Medicine."

He showed me a sheet with a Latin inscription on it. I recognised it straight away. It was a prescription for a peppermint mixture, a harmless antacid you might take for your stomach. The chemist knew to give the patient a pint bottle of this white liquid and they thought they had the cure for whatever ailed them. Over the years, as things changed, I noticed doctors weren't giving as many prescriptions out and didn't spend as much time with their patients, who often came out disgruntled after their appointment and grumbling, "He said nowt and I got nowt." People have to come out feeling either that you've talked to them and led them somewhere or given them something they need. That was a real pearl of wisdom from Dr John that many GPs could learn from today.

Being a locum GP in Leeds was hard work, especially at night. The girls on the switchboard would give me my instructions and I'd drive through the night to see patients. At three o'clock one morning I was bombing across the city to get to a woman who had gone into labour in the block of flats where she lived. There was no traffic around so I put my foot down – until I saw the blue lights flashing in my rear-view mirror. The officer was just getting ready to read the riot act when I got in my defence first, explaining that I was a doctor on my way to deliver a baby. So they followed me all the way and parked outside the flats to give me protection! I had to work in the dark because the electricity meter inside the flat had been cut off. I was on my knees on the floor with this poor woman on the edge of the bed as she gave birth. Afterwards I stitched her up by torchlight and then left her a note for her own doctor saying the baby had been born without any complications.

"Everything all right, Doc?" asked the officer as I walked back out carrying my bag.

"All's well," I nodded.

"That's good. But next time, please don't drive so fast!"

9

Life in General

We spent three and a half years in Leeds and I loved it. But the chance to come home was one I couldn't miss. When a job came up as senior registrar for the North East Rotation I decided to apply for it. I was interviewed at the Northern Region Hospital Board in Newcastle and was successful. Senior registrar was the step below consultant. In those days you did it for anywhere from two to five years or even longer. I wasn't attached to one hospital but worked at three of the largest hospitals in the region, Middlesbrough General, Sunderland and Newcastle. At Middlesbrough General I worked with some really good old fashioned surgeons who all had extensive wartime experience. Gilbert Parker was the senior man, Matt Leitch was number two, then there was Bruno Isserlin and Dougal Caird. At Sunderland I worked for Adrian Bain, who was sports doctor and surgeon for the British Athletic team. As it was the centre of the region, I had a teaching session at Newcastle every week to keep abreast of developments. It was here that I began to hone my joint replacement skills.

When a consultant's job came up at Middlesbrough General Hospital, Gilbert rang me and told me to apply. I knew that when you get a call like that they must want you. But to my disappointment, I didn't get it. Instead, it went to a Scotsman called Sandy Birnie, who was a couple of years older than me. I carried on in my rotation until another post came up a year later. Once again Gilbert invited me to apply. This time I was up against a man

I'd known from Leeds, David Heath. We were both interviewed and I got the job. In those days before trusts, I was appointed by Newcastle Regional Health Authority. On my way back home to Middlesbrough I stopped at a service station on the A1 and rang Freda to tell her the good news. By now she was teaching at St Thomas's Secondary School in Middlesbrough but she also helped out at her sister Ena's shop in North Ormesby on evenings and weekends. We arranged to meet a couple of doors down from there at Norman Baum's Cafe. We celebrated our good news in style – with a cup of tea and an iced bun!

My colleagues at Middlesbrough General were a great bunch. Once again I was back working with men who'd taught me, Gilbert Parker and Dougal Caird, but now I was a Consultant Orthopaedic Surgeon alongside them. Together with Matt and Bruno we made a formidable gang. They were all great men. Gilbert and Dougal were an inspiration to everybody. Gilbert looked after me like a son, even though he had one of his own. Matt was a dear Irishman who I also have very fond memories of. There were also some excellent general surgeons, including Frank Graham and Jimmy Oldfield, who was still based at North Ormesby. It was always good to see Jimmy. I'd ring him if I had someone with an injury such as a ruptured bladder and he always said how old I made him feel.

"I remember you when you were training and now you're working alongside with me as a colleague," he'd laugh. But if Jimmy felt old, how must Matt have felt? He'd looked after me as a boy when I'd had my back problem. Matt and the others were getting on in years and as their health began to wane I was often left on my own. I put a lot of hours in during those early days. There was no question of getting locums in – you just got on with it and did the work yourself.

Everyone had a tremendous work ethic. There was a great team throughout the hospital and everybody helped each other. If Patrick Clark, an excellent neurosurgeon, was going away for the weekend, he'd ask me to look in on his department for him. If there were any problems I'd call him so he could guide me through them. That wouldn't happen these days but Patrick knew I'd experienced that kind of situation during my time in the RAF. I was once on call and went in at three in the morning to put a lad's leg back together after it had been mangled in a motorbike accident. As I was walking in, I saw Gilbert walking out.

"What have you been up to?" I asked.

"Oh, I've just stitched somebody's heart up after he got stabbed down the town."

The thought of an Orthopaedic Surgeon stitching someone's heart up would seem very odd to a young surgeon today. But because Gilbert had done that kind of thing in the war he was used to it. If someone has a puncture wound in the heart you open the chest and put your finger on it while you put a couple of stitches in. Nowadays people with that kind of injury wouldn't survive if there wasn't the right specialist around, because nobody else would touch it. But that's what it was like back then, especially with surgeons who had been in the forces. They were used to doing things guys training today never get the chance to do. I was of the post-War generation but many of my colleagues had worked throughout World War II. One of them, Frank Walker, saw action at Arnhem as a doctor in the Paras.

When lads become consultants now they don't have anything like the experience we had. My training career was opening chests, heads, spines, everything. Now you do a four-year course as a trainee and whizz around various hospitals and see bits and pieces of different specialities. Within orthopaedics you might see a few children's cases and joint replacements, but you don't really spend time there or actually *do* very much for yourself. That means that when they're appointed, they often have very little practical operative experience. Our training was more of an apprenticeship, where we actually learned to do things ourselves.

When I met the Army's Director of Medical Training I told him he needed to send all his trainees out to Afghanistan for six weeks. That short time would make a massive difference throughout the rest of their careers. Doctors are pretty safe in the hospitals over there, they don't get attacked very often. They would see everything, including more trauma cases than they would in a lifetime over here, and it would stand them in good stead. The art and science of surgery only really advances during wartime. During the First and Second

World Wars we learned a huge amount about the infection of wounds and fractures to bones. If you got a broken femur in the old days, you were dead. Then the Thomas splint came out and changed everything. It was a metal calliper that enabled the leg to be straightened and bandaged tightly, which would keep it safe. It was invented by Hugh Owen Thomas, who is sometimes called the father of orthopaedic surgery in Britain. He worked in Liverpool in the nineteenth century, but his contribution to medicine was never fully appreciated in his lifetime. The splint was introduced during World War I by Thomas' nephew, Sir Robert Jones, dramatically reducing the mortality rate from fractures to the femur. You cleaned up the wound, wrapped the leg and then the patient could be transported home. The technique was developed further during World War II at Tobruk in North Africa, where soldiers had been blown apart by tank shells. To prevent the damaged limb from being jolted around as field ambulances crossed the rough desert terrain, the leg and splint were padded and then encased in Plaster of Paris. This became known as the Tobruk splint. There were further advances during the Korean War and again in Vietnam. There we learned about resuscitation and getting people to medical facilities as soon as possible, while ensuring they were given fluid. Pour fluid in and get them into a helicopter as soon you can. Afghanistan has taught us yet more lessons. We've learned with multiple injuries to replace the fluid they've lost, stop any bleeding, push the organs back in and bandage the patient up, instead of spending all night trying to put things back together. Get them stabilised and the next morning, when the blood pressure's up again and the heart's normal and the electrical-chemical factory seems to be reasonably normal, then they're fit to go theatre. If you operate when they're not fit that's when they die, either under the anaesthetic or soon afterwards. When I was a young man, if I got someone who'd been pulled in off the A19 with a mangled leg from a motorcycle accident, I'd be up all night putting the leg back together. Now we know that's not the way to do it, unless there's an immediate threat to life and limb. If gangrene is setting into his leg, I'd have to go in, find the artery and sort it out and then stabilise the leg so it doesn't bend and tear the repair. Now we know that if you possibly can, you get them fit and well first. I go to the Combined Services Orthopaedic meetings, where young men and women who are surgeons in the forces present papers after they've studied hundreds of cases of bullet wounds through the upper arm. Where else would you get that kind of information? You see veterans on the news with two legs and an arm missing. Twenty years ago they would have died and now they don't. That's directly a result of the experiences we had in Afghanistan. I've always had a great admiration for the pioneers of surgery. I read history books going back to medieval times, fascinated by what the doctors did then. Ambroise Paré was a great French barber surgeon and anatomist in the sixteenth century who learned a huge amount on the battlefield. The science of trauma surgery has always advanced during times of war. I don't think it can advance any further now, I think we've gone as far as we can. What else can we possibly do?

Despite the invaluable lessons my old colleagues had learnt in the war years and even though they were all brilliant trauma surgeons, the treatments available back then were all fairly basic. If you broke your thighbone you lay in a hospital bed at the General on a Thomas splint for two months. If you fractured your tibia you spent three months on a Braun frame or in plaster. The art of internal fixation was in its infancy. In Germany and other parts of the Continent people were beginning to insert plates in tibias and nail down femurs to help repair fractures. Gradually, I began introducing new procedures. One of the first things I was responsible for developing in our region was arthroscopy, inserting a probe into the knee to take cartilage out. I'd picked up the skills in Leeds and I knew they had an expensive, Japanese-made arthroscope gathering dust in a cupboard there because the surgeon who'd been using it had left. Shortly before Christmas one year I told Gilbert we needed to be doing knee arthroscopy and about the unused instrument. He asked how much it would cost. It was £800.

"Right," he said. A few weeks later he dressed up as Santa Claus for the Rotary Club and went round the town collecting the money we needed. Once he had enough I rang Leeds and offered to buy it. It was very primitive compared to the instruments we have now and most of its use was diagnostic. It wasn't fibre-optic and had a tiny light bulb in the end to enable you to see inside the knee. We just put it in and had a look to see how the joint was running. We could take a piece of cartilage out and then get a histologist to have a look at it to see if they could diagnose rheumatoid arthritis. Or we could look in and diagnose a torn cartilage, although we couldn't do anything about it because we didn't have the tools at that time. Operative arthroscopy didn't come in until the 1980s and it's been developing rapidly ever since. These days they even operating on finger joints through mini-scopes.

As well as arthroscopy I'd also developed a major interest in backs during my time in Leeds. I did some of my training with Martin Nelson, who was pioneering new techniques and approaches. He even had a psychologist in his back pain clinic, something I'd never seen before. He believed that you often need a psychologist to help address back pain issues. I thought that was pretty advanced. When I returned to Teesside one of my focuses was on backs, which are a major issue everywhere but especially in an area like ours. In the old days, if a steelworker got a bad back, the doctor wrote out a sick note and ordered physiotherapy treatment and rest. For the rest of their lives these men had exercise and physio once or twice a week. But it didn't cure them and they never returned to work. Instead they all retired on ill health grounds. The whole outlook has changed since then. These days, after a couple of weeks rest, they get you moving and then back to work. You don't wait for the pain to go away, because it won't. If you have some wear and tear in your discs you would have developed backache at some point anyway. The injury has just aggravated it. You'll continue to get some backache – it's natural.

Our treatment for people with acute sciatica in the old days was two weeks bed-rest on traction, as long as there was no definite risk of paralysis. If they were no better after that we injected dye to identify the damaged disc and then whipped it out. Everybody else back then just left it alone until it got better. I once got a call from a surgeon in Newcastle who was an expert in the field and had produced academic papers on orthopaedics. He was such a perfectionist that he had matt black instruments, designed to prevent the light reflecting back off them while he was operating. He wanted to know how many discs I removed and I estimated the figure at about fifty a year –

twenty-five on the NHS and twenty-five privately.

"That's far too many," he said disapprovingly.

Years later, studies came out showing the outcome after two years was the same for patients who had been operated on those who weren't. But you've got to remember that if you don't work for two years, especially in an area like Teesside, you're not earning any money and you're in trouble. Lots of people were self-employed and they just couldn't afford to be off work for two years with sciatica, which is a dreadful, debilitating pain.

I eventually got fed up of bad backs, partly because they don't all get better. You can usually get rid of the terrible pain, but the patient still has some backache and that's life. It's still the same today, nobody cures it all. So I got the system reasonably well organised and then, twenty years ago, I managed to bring in the spinal surgeon Charles Greenhough, who came up from London. I explained to him that Teesside was an industrial area where people needed to be fit for heavy work. I said I wanted him to take the problem of backache by the horns and really tame it. He came back with ambitious plans and developed the Spinal Assessment Unit, staffed by specialist nurses, to see people who GPs referred to us with backache. Bringing in these specially trained nurses was a stroke of genius. If it was just mechanical backache needing strengthening exercises and physio then they could get on with that. If not they were given surgery. It worked very well and was so good that they were invited to go to Australia to tell them how to introduce the system there.

I also started doing joint clinics in partnership with rheumatoid physicians. I was approached with the idea soon after I arrived in Middlesbrough. I'd known Ian Haslock since we were at Leeds together. We were friends and he became a Consultant Rheumatologist in Middlesbrough a year before I was appointed. Rheumatologists were able to prescribe tablets and inject joints, but when their treatment failed the joints would fall to pieces. By running clinics together I could help them decide when they'd gone as far as they were going to get with that approach and a new knee joint was required.

I stayed in that corridor for many years and operated on many of Ian's patients. I'm pleased to see that rheumatology has improved dramatically in recent years and they're often able to treat the problem without surgery now.

But I did countless operations and people were extremely appreciative. They had often spent years with chronic pain in every joint giving them constant problems. Young women in their early thirties would hobble into the clinic doubled up with two bad knees and two bad hips. Afterwards they had their lives back.

"My husband's furious, one woman joked. "He's had to buy me a completely new wardrobe because I'm four inches taller now!"

There's tremendous satisfaction in that. I was able to do something for them that transformed their lives. There are few better feelings in the world than that. I believe it's important to have that relationship with your patients. They have to get to know you and trust you. Nowadays it doesn't always happen that way. It's like being on a conveyor belt in a factory and some surgeons often don't even see their patients again after they've carried out surgery on them. That's such a shame.

10

Fishermen and Friends

"It can't be just work, work, work all the time, John. You're coming salmon fishing with us." Those were the words that heralded my reintroduction to a hobby I hadn't tried out since I was a boy. Back then I took the train to Egton Bridge with a couple of mates to fish for trout on the Esk. I wasn't very enthusiastic about it, but it was a day out. The main attraction was buying a sixpenny packet of Woodbines and smoking them on the riverbank while we waited for a bite. But I'd never been salmon fishing in my life. All I knew what that it's not a poor man's sport. Dougal Caird and Wray Ellis had taken me under their wing in my early days at the General and their offer showed I was now part of the gang. And so, somewhat reluctantly at first, I agreed to join them. They fished the Deveron, a fast-flowing river that went through the town of Huntly in Aberdeenshire. There they met up with two brothers of Seymour Hackett, who was a colleague of ours, an Anaesthetist in Orthopaedics. One of them, Norman, was a gifted fisherman. Norman had been a bank manager in Thurso right up on Scotland's north coast, not far from John o' Groats, and had retired to live in Huntly's old vicarage. The other brother, Peter, was an ex-Army medic who'd become Governor of Peterhead Prison. He didn't fish much but we all met up a hotel in Huntly where we were staying. As soon as we arrived the drinking began – and it continued for the duration of the trip. Each day we'd have a few by the river, a couple on the way home, then a gin and tonic before dinner at Norman's house and wine as we dined. Norman was a great character, a wonderful raconteur and a brilliant historian. Going to his house after dinner in the hotel was part of our daily routine. The first time we went, Wray and Dougal told me Norman would talk all night. But they said that at some point late in the evening his mouth would continue moving and he would stop talking. That, they said, would be our cue to leave. Boy, could Norman drink. But he could take it and it just seemed to make him talk more. He enthralled us all evening with tales about the Highland Clearances and the Jacobite Risings, the attempts to restore the Stuarts to the thrones of England and Scotland in the seventeenth and eighteenth centuries. As well his expertise in history he was steeped in Highland folklore, gripping us with chilling stories of kelpies, the shape-shifting water spirits said to inhabit the lochs and pools of Scotland. Sure enough, just as I'd been told it would, the talking stopped abruptly shortly after midnight. At that point the rest of us quietly slipped away back to our hotel. At seven o'clock the next morning Norman would be there bright as a button, wearing his plus fours and his hat with his bait and a raincoat under his arm. Off we'd go fishing and the drinking would start all over again.

I caught my first salmon on my second trip to the Deveron. It was a tremendous thrill. Norman wasn't fishing that day, but used to ghillie for us, assisting and giving us the benefit of his enormous experience. When I got a bite I called him and he helped me land the fish. There was only one way to celebrate. Norman produced a bottle of whisky and we all had a little nip of Glenfiddich to wet the salmon's head. We only had a tiny dram, so we could get back fishing straight away. When I got another bite I glanced over to the embankment to summon more help. But all I could see was two knees. There was Norman lying flat on his back with his dog alongside him. They were both fast asleep with the bottle of Glenfiddich empty on the grass beside them.

Norman was a great man. But it was his talent as a fisherman that was perhaps his greatest gift. He had an old-fashioned split cane rod, while ours were of a more modern fibreglass construction. When we reached the river in the morning he'd get out of the car and take a quick look over the river and instantly assess our chances for the day.

"Ach, there's nae watter…" was a regular complaint. If that was the case he wouldn't even put his rod up. That was a very bad sign for the rest of us. If Norman wasn't confident of catching anything, we knew we had no hope whatsoever. But we'd try anyway, and whether we caught anything or not we always enjoyed great times together.

When Norman died Wray and Dougal went up for the funeral in Aberdeen. We couldn't all go, so I had to stay at the hospital to hold the fort. Our former colleague Seymour, Norman's younger brother, was also there and it was the only cremation in Aberdeen that day. Seymour and Norman were like chalk and cheese. Norman loved to fish and drank like one as well, while Seymour was a stern and sober member of the Church of Scotland. After the service they all stood there together in the grounds of the crematorium, wondering what they should do next. Someone suggested having a drink at the local club in his memory. At that moment, the smoke started curling out of the chimney and into the steely-grey Scottish sky above.

"Look at that," said Wray, dryly. "You only have to mention booze and Norman's there straight away!"

Seymour wasn't too pleased about his little joke, but it was just the kind of wry humour the rest of us shared together.

I went to the Deveron every spring from the early 1970s onwards. Then, towards the end of every August, we'd go up to the River Oykel, in the far north-west, a few miles inland from Ullapool and on the main road between the east and west of Scotland. It always rains in Scotland and when the rivers flood it's a great time to catch fish. We arrived there one Monday morning at the start of our week and had twelve salmon landed on the bank by lunchtime. All the hotels had big chest freezers to keep the salmon in. We tagged them, wrapped them up in newspaper and brought them home with us. We rarely brought many back. Some people staying in the same hotel as us did, mainly those who were fishing on the expensive part of the river below the bridge. They were MPs, bankers, accountants and judges. They were all great company and the social life in the hotel was brilliant. We were up there when the Guinness scandal was going on and the some of the guys who were involved were there, talking on the phone to their lawyers every day.

The Oykel was beautiful and the part we fished was incredibly cheap as well. We paid about £190 for a week of superb fishing. Down on the fashionable Tweed, a bunch of London bankers would fly up by private jet and pay £4,000 for a weekend on Junction Pool and wouldn't catch a thing. I fished the Oykel with Wray and Dougal every year until, sadly, Dougal became ill and had to stop coming. He suffered a heart attack and subsequently died. After that Wray and I met Jimmy Mitchell, a GP from the Borders area who was a Tweed Commissioner in his spare time. He lived in Paxton, just outside Berwick, and had been born and bred on the banks of the weed. He was in his 70s but was fit as a greyhound and knew everything there was to know about fishing. If he said there were fish over there, you could bet your last half-crown that there were. One time we went and there was no water in the river. There'd been a long, hot, dry spell and there was only a tiny trickle of water wending its way over the rocks. Nobody else caught anything on the whole river all week, but Jimmy always came back with fish. We didn't know how he did it. We suspected he was doing something illegal, but he wasn't; he was just a clever and resolute fisherman.

Over the years the Oykel got very expensive and our old stretch is no longer available to fish on now. The two old ladies who owned it died and it passed on to one of their sons. He put it up for auction and that short piece of the river went for a couple of million quid. Former Harrods owner Mohamed Al-Fayed now owns some of the fishing not far from our old spot and he flies his flag from a castle he bought there. One autumn a couple of years we went with Jimmy up to Thurso, where Norman had lived before retiring to Aberdeenshire. If you go any further up this island than Thurso you'd fall off the end of the world. We stayed in a hotel that was like Fawlty Towers. The owner was a former RAF pilot from Lossiemouth, who had given up flying and decided he wanted to be a hotelier instead. But he hadn't completely adapted to civilian life, it seemed. He kept storming out of the dining room during breakfast, leaving his poor French wife to come out of the kitchen and try to pacify his unhappy guests. Every day they sent us off in the morning with big doorstopper, corned beef sandwiches for our bait. No matter how hungry you got you never really wanted to bite into them. The river was like a canal, dark, black and still, flanked by trees bent over at a sixty-degree angle because of the relentless wind. At night, after we'd finished fishing, we'd go for a walk down to the harbour, where we could see hundreds of salmon jumping out of the water. We knew that as soon as there was a drop of rain on the river they'd be up like a shot.

We had some wonderful times fishing in the Highlands, but it was a long way to go. We would break our journey half way, often at an experimental soft fruit farm run by Dougal's brother-in-law. He worked for the Scottish government and was trying to breed a variety of blackberry that could be picked by machine without being damaged. We'd stay the night there and then get up early and continue on our way.

Later, I joined a syndicate on the Tweed with ten or twelve members, who all paid a set sum every year for the privilege. I fished one Wednesday a month during the season, which doesn't sound like much, but salmon fishing on the Tweed is an expensive pastime. It was just past the bridge at Coldstream and was a beautiful spot with everything you could want, lovely fishing and facilities, including a toilet, which is something you very rarely see on a riverbank. There was even a little cottage you could stay in if you wanted to. But sometimes I was too busy to go and missed my monthly opportunity. Jimmy kept trying to persuade me to give it up. As a Tweed Commissioner he had lots of fishing rights on the river and he would happily take me with him. The last day I went up Jimmy came with me and took me out on a boat. We were opposite a hotel, which had the rights to half the river from their side of the bank, while we had the half from our bank.

"I'll just cruise down here," he said. "Put your line out the back."

Blow me, within fifteen minutes, *whoomf*, I had a big fish on my hook, a sixteen-pounder. I reeled it in and got it into my bag. Five minutes later, *whoomf*, I got another one. This time the line snapped and it got away. It had a knot in it, which had weakened it. But five minutes after that, *whoomf*, I'd got another one.

"Jimmy," I said. "You're asking me to give up fishing here and then you bring me out and give me the best day's fishing I've ever had here!"

Many decent fishermen had spent a year without catching anything. But despite that bumper day, I did give it up. I wasn't ready to put away my rod and tackle altogether, however. When I retired I rang the secretary of the Yorkshire Fly-Fishers' Club over in Cumbria. Wray and Dougal had been members and we sometimes went together at weekends during my younger days. I explained that I was looking for a bit of fishing now I'd retired. He invited me to meet him for coffee at the Eden Bridge Hotel and there he welcomed me to the club.

Fishing's an art. First of all, you have to learn to cast a fly and put it where you want it. You also have to learn the river itself in order to fish it. It's a stalking game. You don't just put your line in and then sit back and watch. You work out where the fish is resting and then try to dangle a fly in front of it. If you're doing it properly, you're up to your chest in water. I couldn't do that nowadays, I'd be swept away. But the problem is that often salmon don't eat. If you kill a trout and open it's stomach up, it's full of half-digested flies. If you gut a salmon there's nothing there, it's empty. They don't feed once they're coming upstream. All they're thinking about is making their way up the river so they can get their fin over! Sometimes you'll be on a bridge and see hundreds of salmon lying beneath the water. But get a juicy fly on your hook and dangle it in front of them and they won't touch it. Fishermen are famous for their tales. Well I won't exaggerate because I don't do that. The biggest salmon I caught was a twenty-pounder on the River Tweed. Most of them are seven-to-twelve pounds and when this one bit I thought I'd caught a nuclear submarine. It just took off, taking me with it. Jack Edmondson, a surgeon from North Ormesby Hospital, was with me and helped bring it in. Even with two of us it was a real fight.

As time went by I started to take my sons, Rich and Eddie, fishing with me. Even though they're both very busy these days we still fish together when we can. Just like me when I was a young doctor being dragged along to the River Deveron by Dougal and Wray, they gave it a go and soon found that they loved it. It's still true what they say in the old angler's maxim – once you catch your first salmon, you're hooked for life.

11

Top Doc

I arrived at Middlesbrough General at a time of great change. Within eighteen months Gilbert had retired from his role as senior surgeon and his deputy Matt followed him out soon afterwards. Even though we were no longer colleagues, we all kept in touch with each other and remained firm friends. Gilbert continued to have drinks at his house every New Year's Day. It was a tradition throughout all the years I knew him and was always a big occasion, attended by every surgeon in Middlesbrough. He lived in a big house at the end of The Grove and had a beautiful conservatory with a real vine growing through it like a tree. I saw them regularly until they died, and then I looked after their wives until they moved away or passed on.

Once the old guard had gone two new men were recruited. David Muckle and Yogish Pai both brought new interests to the hospital. David had done lots of work with children in Oxford and was also involved in professional sport. He eventually worked for FIFA and was the doctor on duty at many of the big football matches throughout the world. After a while we appointed another consultant, Joe Hooley, who very tragically became ill with leukaemia a few years later. He tried every possible treatment, including a bone marrow transplant, but it didn't take and he sadly died. But for a while there were five consultants at the General, Dougal Caird, David, Yogish and myself, and it was a very happy unit. Because we looked after the orthopaedic trauma surgery we were responsible for the A&E Department as well in those early days. I also went over to the paediatric wards to see children who came in with fractures.

I worked hard and took on private and medical-legal work as well. I also did some administrative work, but I was given some good advice from my old boss at North Ormesby, Sam Mottershead. Even when I was a houseman he was getting on in years and a long time afterwards he came to see me with a bad back.

"How are you doing, Anderson?" he asked. "I see you're a consultant now. Can you operate on my back and make it better?"

Sadly, it had got beyond that stage and there wasn't much I could do to help him.

"Are you doing any administration?" he asked as he put his jacket back on after the consultation.

"As little as I can," I told him.

"You do right," he said. "Don't get involved. Get on with your work until you're forty and then spend some time on a few committees."

I tried to heed that advice, keeping my head down as much as possible and getting on with the work I loved. We lived in Nunthorpe for a few years, but Freda and I were both Middlesbrough people. We both fell in love with a house we'd seen in Cambridge Road, Linthorpe. It was a big old Victorian home with a large garden and a beautiful magnolia tree that bloomed in the springtime. When it came up for sale we bought it. Among many things I loved about the house was its location, just a mile from my work at the General. One year in the mid-1970s, when the snow was really bad, I was the only doctor who made it into the hospital. The others lived further out at Great Ayton, Stokesley or Marton and couldn't get in. I just put on my coat and scarf and walked round. The house is full of happy memories for us, mostly because it was always ringing with the laughter of children – and thankfully, it still is.

When I became Senior Orthopaedic Surgeon I was responsible for the administration of the whole department. That meant I had to attend monthly meetings as clinical director representative, reporting on what we'd done and telling them about any problems. I also joined the Orthopaedic Society in the North East. It put on regular social evening where surgeons from the region's five main hospitals, Middlesbrough General, Sunderland, Durham, Newcastle and Cumbria, would meet up every month or so. One of us would give a talk and then we'd have a meal and a few drinks afterwards. It helped keep our education up to date and also enabled us to keep in touch with each other. I became secretary because I always believed that you can't just expect to turn up and not do your bit to help out. That meant organising dinner for twenty-two surgeons at a hotel in Cumbria.

As well as the General we also covered North Tees Hospital, because they only had a couple of orthopaedic surgeons when it opened, Matt Leitch and Wray Ellis. Matt, of course, had been at the General, while Wray had come from Sedgefield Hospital. When North Tees was built they held some operating sessions over there, but they also came over to the General and they were part of our team. Unfortunately, they were both getting on in years. When they were off ill they had no surgeons, so we covered for them. That's another thing you wouldn't get away with these days. I once got a call from North Tees at midnight while I was pinning somebody's leg back together in Middlesbrough.

"We've just received a patient who's been shot in the leg," they said.

"I'll be over as soon as I can," I told them. I finished up what I was doing and headed there straight away.

In 1997 I was appointed Chief of Service for the Trauma Division. My new role involved overseeing plastic surgery, maxillofacial surgery, spinal surgery, ear, nose and throat surgery, A&E and orthopaedics. We had an annual budget of £20m and I was paid about £800 extra per month to take on the additional responsibility. It was a bit like becoming a headmaster who also has his own class to look after. I still had all my own work to do, but everybody else's problems were now mine as well. I'd go in on a Monday morning and find two plastic surgeons on the doorstep of my office after falling out with each other over something or other. It was my job to sort it out. I also had to attend a chiefs' meeting every week. That interfered with my other duties even more. I was working all the hours God sent in the hospital, including night time emergency calls, operating privately in the

Nuffield on Saturdays and doing some medico-legal work as well. Something had to give. I was over sixty by now and decided to give up private practice and let younger lads take do that work. I continued the medico-legal work, knowing I could plan that to suit me.

As the years went on they decided the orthopaedic surgery was getting too busy, so they started bringing in specialist A&E consultants and took that department off us. Some of the new men were ex-Army officers who were very impressive. The first was a Pole, Jarek Kotowski. He was a wonderful character and regaled us with stories from the Second World War. He was surgeon to a Polish cavalry unit that once charged a line of Panzer tanks on horseback with their swords drawn.

"What else could we do?" he said. "We couldn't run away – we were Poles!"

Jarek ran the A&E Department on his own for a few years and then they gradually introduced younger consultants who were doing modern training and developing new forms of treatment. The manager I worked alongside for most of my time as Chief was a great girl called Carol Dargue, who'd been a sister at Hemlington Hospital in my early years. We had an excellent working relationship and have kept in touch ever since.

My working life was an absolute joy and I loved just about every minute. But I had the right people alongside me in a very good team, and that's absolutely crucial. A surgical "firm" is made up of the boss – the consultant – together with a registrar or senior registrar, a trainee registrar and then a houseman. The houseman is responsible for everybody's patients and does some of the day-to-day work, going round to see how they're doing. When the consultant does a ward round it's the junior doctor's job to provide an update on each patient – "Mrs Bloggs had a temperature last night, I've done her bloods and given her antibiotics." Then your trainee would tell you a bit more about what was going on. I was so busy in the first ten to fifteen years after I was appointed as consultant that I refused to take on a senior trainee, because I found it slowed me down so much. You might think that's very selfish, but that's what I did. However, I did have a very good assistant. He was called Tam Zabihi and he was eight years older than me. He had been Assistant Professor of Orthopaedics at the University of Tehran and came from a wealthy family of builders, the Iranian equivalent of Taylor Wimpey. Back home Tam had a stunning collection of luxury cars, from American Cadillacs to Rolls Royces. He owned a collection of hunting rifles and went out shooting in the desert and he also kept stables and raced horses. He was among the most privileged of Iran's wealthy elite. Then, in 1979, came the Islamic Revolution. The Shah, who had ruled for almost forty years, was deposed and the exiled Ayatollah Khomeini was invited back to take power. Tam's parents were placed under house arrest and the new authorities seized everything they owned, including his cars and guns. Tam did some of his medical training in England and married an English ward sister. They had a son and two daughters. Iran quickly became a dangerous place for all of them. The Revolutionary Guard came to the house and made all kinds of grisly threats towards his family. Then Tam returned one day to find his racehorses slaughtered and their heads stuck to the door in true mafia style. Tam didn't need any more warnings after that. He piled everything he could into an estate car and drove his family out of Iran, across Asia and through Europe to the south of France, where he owned a luxury apartment. He still had plenty of money and for a year he did nothing. But as the cash began to dry up he decided he needed to start working again and his wife came up with the idea of returning to England. Even though his knowledge and experience was pretty extensive, no hospital would employ him at anything like the level of seniority he had reached in Iran. Instead he took a job on the lowest rung of the ladder, as a house officer in Darlington. After a while he applied for a job in Middlesbrough. I liked him straight away, although I was also very wary. He was extremely experienced – he even looked after the trauma victims when there was a major earthquake in Iran. Although I could see he was good, much of what he had learned in his homeland belonged to another century. But I decided to take a chance and he came to us as a house officer. He hadn't done the English Fellowship for the Royal College of Surgeons, so he couldn't become a consultant, but I could make him an assistant surgeon. He was delighted. However, for the first ten years he was with me I still did every operation. Tam had a decade of good experience before I let him do an operation for himself. It was a basic hip replacement and I watched over him. He performed it exactly as I did it, move for move, without a stitch out of place, because he'd spent so many years watching me. After that I had a new freedom I'd never enjoyed since I became a consultant. When people have been on a waiting list for two years, the worst thing you can tell them is, "Sorry Mrs Jones, I'm off to France next week and there's nobody else to do your operation, so we'll have to cancel it." Now I could say, "Tam, I'm away next week, this is what I want you to do…" Tam and I became inseparable and he worked with me for the rest of my career until I retired. After that everybody who did private work wanted Tam as their assistant, because they knew he'd been properly trained. Over the next few years he made quite a lot of money as his cut of the surgeons' fees. Some people in the hospital called me "Boss", but to most I was known simply as "Mr A". Tam and I were great friends as well as colleagues and I'd say, "Call me John." But it was always Mr A to Tam. He's in his 80s now and lives in Bristol. Even now when he rings me up he says, "Hello Mr A, how are you?" It's always great to hear from Tam. He was the best assistant I could have wished for.

12

Private Eyes

I didn't become a doctor for the money. I did it to help people get well. Having seen so many children being cured of debilitating illnesses during my time in the Friarage Hospital I decided that was the life for me. Even though I did private work for twenty years, my NHS responsibilities were always of paramount importance to me. During my time we always had a happy knack of appointing people we could get along with. Sometimes I look at people now and wonder how they ever got the job. Once you've appointed someone, of course, it's very difficult to get rid of them. They can play about with their contracts and say they don't want to work eight sessions a week, they only want to work two, to enable them to run off and do private work. Very early on I moved my own private work out to the St John of God Hospital in Scorton, which was run by an order of religious brothers. I worked there every Saturday when I wasn't on call. It was hard work because I often didn't finish my working day until about seven thirty. In the summer I'd pick Freda and the kids up and we'd drive to Scorton, then I'd drop them off on the village green or in the pub. After seeing my patients I'd rejoin the family and we'd have a meal together and then come home. Eventually a long-term plan to develop a private hospital in Middlesbrough came to fruition. Believe it or not, the original idea was to put it on the top floors of the Dragonara Hotel, or Jurys Inn as it is now, in Middlesbrough town centre. That was never going to work – you can't really put a hospital on top of a casino! After that they looked at various sites before settling on on Junction Road in Norton, where they built the Nuffield Hospital. I worked there from its opening until I gave up private practice in 1997. I was also secretary of the medical committee, just to keep an eye on things, and it worked well. In the early days private hospitals didn't have all the facilities needed for the more difficult and risky cases. When they arose the surgeon would contact their own hospital and explain what was going on to his manager. They would then arrange to do the operation in the NHS hospital for an agreed price. That ensured everything was legitimate – because in the early days that hadn't always been the case.

The political climate wasn't always favourable towards private practice when I first started doing it. They began prying to try to find out whether some doctors were treating private patients on NHS property. In about 1980 the NHS sent two accountants to Middlesbrough looking for any abuses that might be going on here. They came into the General and asked who did the most private work. That was the plastic surgeon Charles Viva and me, and so we were the ones who came under scrutiny. They asked my secretary for my private diaries and she told then I didn't have any, because I didn't do any private work there. They weren't having that. They accused her of lying and even threatened her with losing her job. The poor woman was in tears. The same thing happened with Charles. Unlike me, he did his private work at the General. But it was all done on Saturday mornings and properly booked in, listed and above board. Charles had nothing to declare, and because I did all my work at Scorton and then the Nuffield, neither did I. The probe continued for a couple of weeks and when they had completed their enquiries we were all called to a big meeting. Chief executive Bill Murray then gave the accountants an almighty roasting and they were sent home with their tails between their legs. Unfortunately for the snoopers they'd picked on the wrong blokes. They could have chosen ten other surgeons and ended up clapping their hands with glee. I once heard about an NHS surgeon telling a junior doctor in his firm to bring a couple of standard Charnleys to the Harley Street clinic where he was doing private work. That meant they were effectively stealing. There was a lot of abuse like that in other parts of the country. And I've got to say that some North East surgeons weren't averse to it either.

My involvement in sports injuries began when I was at the General but its roots went back to my time in Sunderland. My boss when I was a senior registrar on the North East Rotation there was Adrian Bain, who looked after the British Olympic team as well as a number of Rugby League clubs in South Yorkshire, including Wakefield Trinity, Castleford and Huddersfield. When he was dying Adrian left instructions with the clubs to contact me if they had any problems. Within a week of him passing away, the phone rang.

"Doc, we've got two players with ligament injuries," said the voice on the other end of the line.

That was the start of a long and very enjoyable association with the sport. The Wakefield chairman would often bring a player up in his car on a Monday morning after they'd picked up an injury in the weekend's game. I'd see them as soon as I could and then operate either that afternoon or the next week.

Then the Newcastle and Gateshead Harriers athletics club found out what I was doing and they started coming down to see me. The athletes always seemed to bring their wives with them. When anyone asks if they can bring their wife, I always say I don't mind if you don't – but you might have to tell me few little secrets they don't know about! That always gets a laugh. Many of these athletes were addicted to running. When they were out of action because of an injury, the wives would say, "For God's sake Doctor, sort him out, because he's driving me mad!"

There are various groups of prima donnas in the world. Athletes are bad, and fighter pilots aren't much better, but footballers are undoubtedly the worst of them. When they get little aches and pains they want them sorting out instantly. I became involved with Middlesbrough Football Club when one of my colleagues decided to give up the role because it was too demanding and didn't pay enough. The club doctor, Laurie Dunn, rang me up and said he had a player down in Hull who had broken his leg. They sent him up and I nailed his tibia, a procedure we'd recently started doing. It enabled players to return to the game much more quickly than they had previously been able to. They were impressed and started sending me more players who were having problems. Two great lads I operated on were the goalkeeper, Stephen Pears, who was having trouble with tendonitis in his calves, and the striker, Bernie Slaven. Bernie was actually the last player I did for the club. It was shortly before a game they needed to win to get into the Premier League. He'd torn his cartilage and it had to come out. I removed it with an arthroscopy and he was back playing in three weeks. He went on to score the goals that won Boro promotion, so I must have done a decent job. But the club sometimes took their time to settle their bills. They seemed to think I should see it as an honour to look after their players, rather than my job. We had a few arguments and in the end I decided I'd had enough, just like the previous man had.

I also gave up working with the rugby clubs in the early 1980s, because it was becoming too time-consuming. An A&E doctor in Wakefield who was interested in sport became involved with the club. After a while I suggested that he should take it over on his own and he agreed. But I had some memorable experiences during my time with them. I went down to watch games and they were lovely people. Rugby League is very different from football, with much more of a family atmosphere. You could take your kids to the matches and the Yorkshire people were so friendly, passing round cups of tea and sandwiches to the kids. Wakefield Trinity reached the Rugby League Cup final at Wembley and invited me down to the game with my family and I was on the touchline and giving the players injections at half-time to keep them going. My boys loved that.

I was happy to give up private practice when I was appointed Chief in 1997. Some people said I must be daft. The NHS didn't pay particularly well and I just got the basic orthopaedic surgeon's salary. You might get a merit award if they thought you were very good. Before he retired Wray Ellis put my name down for an award of around £6,000 a year extra. Those accountants didn't find any abuses because with Charles and I there weren't any. That wasn't because we thought anyone was watching us. It was what we believed was the right thing to do. You can't fiddle the NHS. If you do, those who can't afford to pay privately are the ones who suffer. Some of the patients I saw had waited two years for an operation – and they had the right to get it when we'd told them they were going to get it. I'll tell you a story that sums up the prevailing attitude in my team. One Christmas Eve, things ran over in the operating theatre and everybody was harassed. Understandably, the theatre staff wanted to finish as soon as possible and get home to be with their families. We had one more operation to do, a hip replacement.

"I think we should cancel the last case," I said.

But my anaesthetist wouldn't hear of it.

"Look," he said. "This poor bugger has waited eighteen months for this operation and I think he should get it."

I knew he was right.

"So do I," I said. And despite the disruption it caused for them and their families, every one of the theatre staff agreed. That's what they were like in those days. If it needed to be done, they'd do it. I'm not sure that's always the case now.

13

To Pastures New

The General was a great place and I loved it. But for many years there had been proposals to build a new hospital to serve the people of Teesside. At one time they were going to put it where Middlesbrough Football Club's Riverside Stadium is now. However, a preliminary examination of the site revealed that it was toxic because of an old chemical works that had been there. Instead South Cleveland Hospital was built on Marton Road in 1980. I wince when I think of the billions of pounds that will have to be paid back in the next few years under the terms of the Public Finance Initiative the hospital was built under.

Even back then I could foresee the traffic problems that the big new hospital would bring. The renal physician David Kenwood telephoned me when he was chair of the Area Medical Committee.

"If you were to come over to the South Cleveland site, what would you want most of all?"

I thought about it for a moment.

"A parking spot with my name on it right beside the front door," I said.

It was just a joke at the time, but you wouldn't believe the battles we had about parking in the years that followed – and they're still going on today!

Hemlington Hospital, where I enjoyed many happy years, had closed down a year earlier as part of the restructuring of local services. Most trauma cases were dealt with at Middlesbrough General, while elective surgery, such as joint replacements and routine spine ops, were usually carried out at Hemlington. We were all very sad to see it go. It was designated as one of the hospitals that would receive casualties from the D-Day landings in 1944. They expected thousands of wounded soldiers and planned to bring them back across the Channel and send them to emergency hospitals around the country. Gilbert Parker was responsible for preparing Hemlington as part of the plans. It was little more than a series of wooden huts, but it served us well for years until it closed. I did thousands of operations there and I loved it. They demolished the building not long after it closed.

When it first opened, the new hospital didn't include Orthopaedics or a Casualty Department. We remained at Middlesbrough General until the last minute. The surgeons moved out first, so we took over their beds in one of the newer blocks at the General, giving us some extra space. A few years later, in the summer of 2003, we followed them. In the end our hands were forced and we made the move a few months earlier than we planned to. The decision was hastened by a chance event and a decision by our chief executive, Bill Murray. When the powerhouse flooded the whole of Middlesbrough General was without power – and without power, we couldn't function. We found ourselves in a dangerous place and Bill decided we should take the hint.

"Right," he said. "We're moving."

Bill was a key cog in a very good team. I enjoyed a good relationship with him and we worked well alongside each other. The whole set-up was highly successful. Within a couple of days we'd packed up and gone. We loved the old place so much that someone came up with the idea of the staff marching to the new site together as a mark of respect. So we did. About 100 of us took part in the two-mile procession and my two little granddaughters were pictured in the *Evening Gazette* dressed as nurses.

One of the biggest differences that struck us when we first arrived at South Cleveland was how new and clean everything was. But it was hard work adapting to our new surroundings. We found ourselves in an unfamiliar environment, while staff from other departments were already firmly embedded in theatre. We only took a few of our own nurses and everything moved very slowly. The procedures that had served us so well and made everything so efficient were no longer in place. The huge size of the complex meant it took forever to get patients to theatre. That was a major bugbear with me. A surgeon wants to finish an operation and find the next patient ready in the anaesthetic room. I wasted hours twiddling my thumbs in between operations instead of getting on with the next patient straight away as I was used to. Not that I rushed things. I always talked to patients before they were put to sleep.

"How are you doing? Which leg are we chopping off today?" That was a joke I often used, but it also served to focus your attention.

Little things like seeing patients before surgery and again as they're waking up are important. People really got to know and trust you because you had that close working relationship with them. But sadly they don't always do it like that nowadays. I read medical reports where people have had operations and the level of care we gave just isn't there anymore. It grieves me when I think how hard I worked to show my boys how to do things properly. People I trained tell me they try to do things the way I taught them, but are restrained from doing so by red tape. Today's NHS is constantly looking over every consultant's shoulder to see how they measure up against targets. If you're seeing more returning patients than new patients you get into trouble. That's not the way I was brought up. When you treated somebody you followed them up until they were better. Sadly, you're not allowed to do that nowadays. That's one of the reasons I wouldn't be happy working in the NHS now.

Fortunately, however, some of the customs I helped establish at South Cleveland continue today at what is now the James Cook University Hospital. Andy Port, who we appointed as a consultant and is now Chief, has carried on the old fashioned traditions of personal care. He's excellent. If anybody has a hip replacement that goes wrong he can fix it because he was taught right. He watched me, learned from me and looked after patients just as I did. He's improved many procedures and introduced improved clinical methods, but at the same time he's retained the right way of caring for patients.

As well as the delays, we didn't have enough space in those early days. I'd been involved in advising on what the new Orthopaedic Unit should look like and when they designed it I told them it was too small. As medical practices changed, however, we didn't need as much space as we once did. When a motorcyclist broke his leg he used to spends three months in a splint. Now he gets it pinned back together and is home in five days. That meant we no longer needed all the beds we once did. The same happened in other clinical areas. When I was a child I spent all those months in a spinal frame at Northallerton. As we gained more confidence and technology improved, turnaround times reduced dramatically.

As the months passed by we began to settle into our new surroundings. We brought up any problem we were experiencing at committees and one by one they were ironed out. During that time I was able to develop various units, giving them their own autonomy and gradually enabling them to manage themselves. We carried on developing the service. Even though I had a fantastic relationship with my manager Carol, we also had a few run-ins. When they came under government pressure to meet targets they would sometimes steal patients from the end of my waiting lists and send them to be treated privately by someone else. That irritated me because you can run into problems when you do that. I'd end up seeing them a year later with bent, stiff knees after a joint replacement that had gone wrong. It also meant that I lost that personal touch with my patients. I was annoyed about that and let them know.

But over the years we went from strength to strength. I was very proud to play a part in our successful bid for the regional spinal unit. We were up against stiff competition from Newcastle and Sunderland who both wanted it on their sites. Winning that was a major step forward. As we put together our bid I was able to use my contacts to estimate how many cases we would need to treat over a year. The chief exec and medical director could then work out the sort of facilities we would need. Charles Greenhough, now Professor Greenhough, the man I appointed as spinal surgeon twenty years ago when I didn't want to do back surgery anymore, is now in charge of the unit. It's now a world leader in its field and looks after patients from the Scottish borders in the south to Cumbria in the west and Scarborough in the east. There's nothing comparable between Glasgow and Wakefield. Anybody who suffers a broken spine in this area is brought here by ambulance or flown into the helipad at James Cook.

We recruited some extra consultants including a back surgeon, a paediatric surgeon and a hand surgeon. I think we took three or four from North Tees Hospital up the road in Stockton. I didn't poach them, but they'd been our trainees and were keen to return "home". The tradition of former trainees getting consultant jobs elsewhere but eventually coming back to the mothership continues today. Paul Gregg was a trainee of ours from the old Hemlington days who became a Reader in Edinburgh and Professor of Orthopaedic Surgery in Newcastle. I thought he wanted to come back to Middlesbrough so I put a plan together and made him an offer he couldn't refuse. By then he was president of the British Orthopaedic Association and on lots of committees and working closely with the government. Having someone like that who has their finger on the pulse of what's going on can be invaluable. I asked him to do five sessions for us and he could do whatever he wanted with the other five sessions. Tony Unsworth, the Professor of Engineering at Durham, made him a Professor of Orthopaedic Engineering and Paul retired two years after me.

As I came towards retirement there was an increasing shortage of available beds and, more importantly for me, of operating lists. Some guys were lucky if they got one or two lists a week. That's no good. Surgeons should have three or four operating lists a week and maybe a couple of clinics as well, one to see new patients and one to review old ones. At the same time as the operating lists were shrinking the Trust took over the running of the Friarage Hospital at Northallerton again. They had spare beds and operating times, but at first the Trust management couldn't get anyone to go down there to work. As Chief you lead by example and I was very happy to do so. I went to Northallerton to check it out and found everything to be shipshape. Many of the staff were ex-services and I quickly formed a very good relationship with them. Army medics bring that military discipline with them into the hospitals they join after they leave the forces. In some ways it functioned like a military hospital. So as well as continuing to work at James Cook I started doing one or two lists a week at the Friarage. I was free on Thursday afternoons and no longer did any private work. For a while it was difficult to get others to come down with me from James Cook, but eventually I persuaded them. Some were reluctant to take on the extra work. In the modern NHS people sometimes do the minimum required of them. If they're asked to do anything over and above that, they hold their hands out for more money. I had to tell a few people that they were employed on a nine-session contract and had only done eight sessions. I agreed to would pay their travel expenses, but that was all.

I thoroughly enjoyed my time at the Friarage. It has a special place in my heart because of my time as a patient in the children's ward. I can still clearly recall lying in bed one dark night as a thunderstorm raged outside. A tree just near the window was struck by lightning and exploded into flames. The stump stayed there for years. I went back into my old ward one night when I was working at the hospital. The nurses were having a break and were surprised to see me coming in. They almost dropped their plates!

"I used to be a patient in this ward," I told them.

I walked in and there it was at the end of the row on the left-hand side.

"I was in that bed for nine months," I said.

I was Chief for about eight years until I retired in 2005. I didn't want to stop doing what I loved, but the time had come. I still have many, many friends at James Cook and keep in touch with them. Whenever someone retires or there's a celebration, they always ring me up and it's great to meet up and see the old faces.

There are about twenty-eight consultants at James Cook now and there have been many other changes. Morale has fallen and it's not the happy team it once was. When I was made Chief of Trauma in 1997 I was a shop-floor sort of guy. I went to the meetings every week and let them know about our problems, but I remained very much hands-on. You can't treat people at arm's length from an office and just send out messages like some kind of faceless manager. You have to go out and see them face to face and I was constantly going round the place. I'd visit the wards every few days to see where the problems were. There was a very close camaraderie between all of us.

When the outbreak of Mad Cow Disease meant that all surgical instruments had to be double cleaned, operating lists were delayed as a consequence. Surgeons couldn't get the instruments they needed and some of them reacted by shouting and swearing at the girls in the Central Sterile Services Department, whose job it was to provide them. The girls weren't happy and were even talking about going on strike because of the abuse they were experiencing. When I went down for a chat with them I'd take a box of Kit Kats in with me to share round. Funnily enough I always seemed to get my instruments first! It was such a simple gesture, but far more effective than shouting and swearing will ever be. They were so appreciative and they never forgot it. Not long ago, some girls came up to me and Freda in a restaurant.

"It's Mr Anderson, isn't it?" one of them said. "We remember you – and we remember your Kit Kats!"

14

Hip Service

Hip surgery has been one of the most important advancements in the last fifty years. As a young doctor I could see the way we were going and it was incredibly rewarding to be able to develop these exciting procedures in our area. In the couple of years before I arrived there'd been about twelve hip and knee joints done in Middlesbrough by various surgeons having a go at the new techniques. By the end of my time I was doing that many in a good week!

Wrightington, in Lancashire, was the birthplace of hip replacement surgery. It was there that John Charnley, later to become Sir John, set up his base. Along with Kenneth McKee, in Norwich, Sir John was one of the pioneers of artificial joint replacement. As well as being a brilliant and incredibly inventive surgeon, Charnley was also a gifted engineer. He did extensive research into the idea of hip replacement, basing all his work on the low friction principle. His aim was to find two surfaces that could move very well against each other without wearing out.

When he started off in the early 1960s Charnley made the cups we use to hold the joints in place out of polytetrafluoroethylene. Better known by the trade name Teflon, the material was discovered by DuPont in the USA in the 1930s and had been used in the Manhattan Project, which led to the development of the atomic bomb. Teflon was the in thing and was being used in all kinds of household items and famously in non-stick pans. One of its key qualities was how well it facilitated low-friction movement. After a month being tested in a simulator the joint was still working fine. When Charnley put it into people, however, it wore out within a couple of years. That meant he had to take out his first 400 replacement hips and do them all over again. Charnley went back to the drawing board. He approached the chemical giant ICI, who were the experts in plastics, and told them about his research. He asked if they could produce a new, hard plastic for a cup he could fit a metal head into. But ICI were too busy researching other things and weren't interested. Instead he visited the Rhurchem plastics works during a trip to visit some colleagues in Germany. While he was in there he picked up some shavings off the floor and then brought them home and analysed them. The material was known as High Molecular Weight Polyethylene (HMWP) and was similar to the material they make household washing-up basins from, but of far higher density. It had the lowest friction coefficient of any substance he could find. If a material has a high coefficient of friction it puts a strain on the fixation of the cup and it will eventually loosen when the hip moves. But if the material is low-friction, and the cup is well cemented in place, it will last far longer. With HMWP the wear was incredibly low – just 0.1 millimetres every year if it was properly put in. HMWP became the plastic used in the first successful Charnley hip – and ICI missed out on a fortune. Charnley's followers formed the Low Friction Society to continue his work. I've got the society's tie, with its emblem of the Greek letter *Mu*, which is used in classical physics and engineering to represent the coefficient of friction.

Since I was first appointed in the 1970s I've had Charnley's maxim etched on my brain. It was something he drummed into me and all his students. Every Christmas, the RSPCA reminds us that a dog is for life. When it comes to hip joint replacements, the same principle applies. A hip joint is for life. You've put it in, and if anything goes wrong with it, you're responsible for sorting it out. That's why I always thought careful follow up was so important. That way you got to know how things worked. You learn about common issues to look out for. Back then there was nobody to come and sort things out for you – nobody else had the training to do it. Of course I could always ring up Wrightington if I was having a problem I couldn't solve myself. One of the surgeons there, perhaps Mike Wroblewski or John Murphy, would say, "Yes, we've had that problem, this is what you need to do…" That's how you learn. We spent a day operating with Sir John and then a day in his clinics. He had operated on thousands of people and he had assistants to help, but every single patient for the first twenty years or so was seen every year in that clinic. They would have an x-ray and a little chat so he could assess his own results and understand exactly what was going on. So having been trained that way, I naturally did the same thing. After about a decade of operating my orthopaedic review clinics were huge. I might have a hundred patients to see. But after a while we developed a speedy process.

"Hello, Mrs Jones, how are you doing?"

"Oh, it's great, Mr Anderson."

Then I'd look at the x-ray and if everything seemed to be all right I'd arrange to see them again in another year. I thought it was vital to do that, but eventually the numbers got out of hand and I needed some help. I gave a talk to the local GPs in the late 1980s and said it would cost them £25,000 a year for two sisters to run the unit for me. I told them they didn't have the time to do it themselves – and that, with respect, they didn't have the expertise either. They agreed to pay for them and together we developed the arthroplasty practitioner role. The idea was for a senior nurse to be trained for three months, following me around my clinics and getting to know what the x-rays looked like and learning about the major symptoms patients experienced. If patients had unexplained pain they could ring her up and she could examine them. The system worked very well and it gave people confidence. If there was anything she couldn't deal with the sister would just knock on my door and ask me to take a look at the x-ray. The GPs paid for a few years, but then the funding dried up and the NHS wouldn't pay either.

Over my career I replaced thousands of joints, more hips than knees. I honestly couldn't tell you how many I've done in total. When we first moved to James Cook and were struggling to get things organised I sometimes only had two operating sessions a week. As time went on vacant theatres became available and the number of sessions increased. At one point I was offered eight sessions a week, virtually two every working day – and I had my clinics and other work to do on top of that. Tam and I got through 400 hip operations between us that year. I told the junior doctor on our firm to look closely at all 400 patients and list any complications they suffered – such as immediate post-orthopaedic bleeding or thrombosis – so we could assess how we were doing. I've still got the paper he produced and it continues to form the basis of our knowledge at James Cook. When patients ask what the possible complications are you can tell them there's a one per cent chance of damaging their sciatic nerve, a three percent chance of a dislocation, and so on. We know that because we studied our actual results. That's really what the National Joint Register does nowadays, but it's able to do it on a much bigger scale. That was an unusual year, but I would have done three or four a week on average for most of my career.

My patients were very happy and I still see some of them around town today. It's hugely rewarding to know I've made a difference to their lives. I was in the supermarket recently and a man hobbled up to me.

"It's Mr Anderson, isn't it?" he said.

I gave him my standard response when a stranger asks me that question.

"It might be," I smiled.

"You did my hip forty-two years ago," he told me.

I couldn't be that old, I thought.

"Are you sure it's forty-two years ago?" I queried. He was absolutely certain. He was only thirty-five at the time and had developed an arthritic hip that was crippling him.

"I couldn't walk and I couldn't work, and you replaced it for me," he explained.

"Is it still going strong?" I asked.

"Yes," he said. "And I'm seventy-seven now."

It had dislocated a couple of times, which is to be expected because the plastic wears out over forty years, but he was still getting around perfectly well on it.

Another time a man in his fifties came along for an appointment for his elderly mother, who had fallen and broken her hip.

"I had to come with my mam today because I wondered if you would remember me," he said.

I had to admit, I didn't.

"I was doing some welding in a bucket high up off Saltburn pier when the acetylene bottle exploded," he said. "I was on fire and the mechanism melted, so the bucket couldn't be lowered to bring me back down. I jumped over the side and fell thirty feet onto the sand. My foot and my ankle were in a right mess – and you put it all back together."

"How is it now?" I asked.

"Fine," he replied.

That makes you feel good. There's an old joke between physicians and surgeons. We say physicians just write prescriptions and give out tablets and then when they don't work they send their patients to us surgeons. But the truth is we're fortunate that we're able to see our results in a very dramatic way. The first time I meet a patient he or she may be in agony and five days later when you've operated on them they're sorted for another thirty years.

I was talking to a new consultant surgeon who had recently arrived in Middlesbrough.

"You're Mr Anderson," he said.

"Might be," I said as I shook his hand.

"You won't remember me, but I was a houseman fifteen years ago," he said, before explaining that he did foot and ankle surgery.

"I've just seen a patient you operated on nine years ago," he said.

"How is it?" I asked.

"Brilliant," he told me. That's what you like to hear. They can't all be like that. I know there'll be others that will fall out after a year or so. But in general, it's all about the way you do it.

In later years, I brought younger men in as consultants who'd been trained to do shoulders and elbows. That meant I could concentrate mainly on hips and knees. But in the early days I'd get people coming in with terrible elbow problems or permanently stiff shoulders and I wanted to do something to help. If I didn't do it nobody else could – and that would have condemned the patient to a lifetime of pain. So I went to Edinburgh University Hospital to learn elbow operations from Willie Souter, who, like me, did rheumatoid surgery and was the best in the business when it came to elbows. When I arrived another doctor greeted me.

"If you've come to see Mr Souter I hope you've brought your lunch," he said.

I asked what he meant, but he just laughed.

He was meticulous and took four hours to do each elbow. But he did a beautiful job and his results were fantastic. I remember thinking, "I don't have four hours to spare to do an elbow joint!"

But in fact, I managed to do them more quickly and got even quicker as time went by and I gained more experience.

It was a similar story with the ankle. The first operation out was called the STAR ankle, the Scandinavian Total Ankle Replacement. Again, I went a couple of times to Edinburgh and a surgeon came over from Scandinavia to show us how it was done. It was just like being a young surgeon again. I'd watch a couple of operations in the morning, assist with a couple in the afternoon and then do one on my own before I came home and started doing them here.

I also went abroad to develop my skills with shoulders and ankles. In the early days, back in the 1970s, I visited the ENOD-Klinik in Hamburg. They had made advances in dealing with infection in joints, which is always a problem. Nowadays it's even worse with all these antibiotic-resistant organisms. If we were unlucky enough to get an infection back then we would meticulously remove it all, fill it with antibiotics, leave it for three months and then go back in. But the Germans developed new techniques and I made sure I learned from them.

I consider myself extremely lucky to have used the right joints and been trained personally by Sir John Charnley. You've got to learn properly from the right people. And invariably, in my experience, the guy who develops the technique or the device is the best man to teach you. You might have to travel to France, Italy or Germany, but it's worthwhile. If you just read something out of a book you can think something sounds brilliant. Then the manufacturer will send you a video and you watch it and think, "I can do that!" But it's just not the same as getting first-hand advice. You need to talk to the guy, ask him questions and find out what problems he's had. I would go anywhere I could to improve my knowledge and make sure I did my job to the highest standards that I possibly could. That's always been my ethos and it's served me well.

15

Sir John's Legacy

The standard Charnley Hip came onto the market in 1962 and was patented for twenty-five years. It was a huge step forward and has transformed thousands of lives. But the week the patent ended, other firms started producing their own versions. Some completely unsuitable replacement joints came out. Reps would come round offering to send surgeons to New York if they agreed to buy their new products. A lot of that went on. I tried out six imitation Charnley-style joints, but I wasn't satisfied with any of them.

"It's not a Charnley," I told my assistant, Tam, about each one in turn. "It just doesn't feel like a Charnley."

It turned out to be a wise decision. A year later all hell broke loose. Thousands of these new joints all over the world started failing. As a surgeon who was among the most active in the field at this time I was asked to be a witness in some of the lawsuits that followed. My role was to examine all the cases in the West Indies. They sent me hundreds of x-rays to assess and I had to determine whether the surgeon or the joint was at fault. It was six of one and half-a-dozen of the other. A lot of the surgery wasn't good, but there were design faults with the hips as well. The imitations were cheaper and some just weren't made from suitable materials or to the right quality standards. Since those first joints were developed, hundreds more have flooded onto the market.

It was the same story with knee joints. In the 1980s, I attended a knee replacement conference in London, along with my colleague, Dougal Caird. There were 350 different designs of knee on offer and you could take your pick. I was extremely lucky. I chose a mechanically-sound hip joint and used it for most of my surgical career. It worked perfectly, while many others failed within a year or two. In tests on rigs they worked perfectly. But there was little understanding of the biomechanical forces at work in the body during everyday use.

The original Charnley hip was a work of genius. The design was brilliant and it's still working well today for many, many people. But it's important to continue trying to improve the technology and reduce some of the problems that can arise. In a normal hip replacement the surgeon chops the head off the thigh bone and throws it away. A metal stem with a metal head is applied using cement or an alternative fixative. You then place it into the plastic socket, or cup, and you've got the basic replacement hip. But some joints have snapped and surgeons are always asking questions to see if they can improve things. Using principles of physics and mechanics Sir John Charnley calculated that the ideal diameter for the head was twenty-two millimetres. That meant the early heads were relatively small, made from twenty-two millimetres of cobalt-chrome-molybdenum steel. Their small size also made them more prone to dislocate, however. People started asking whether it would be possible to make the head slightly bigger, so it wouldn't dislocate as often. They also experimented with stronger steels to improve the design further.

A friend of mine, Derek McMinn, wanted to find the answer to another question. He asked why we couldn't just cover the head with a metal cup and put a metal socket in so that the joint was metal on metal. That means there's no stem, making it easier to put right if the joint fails. You've only attached the head so you can still chop it off and put a standard hip in later. Derek perfected the design, which was called Birmingham Hip Resurfacing. It was excellent and around 95% of them are still working well ten years on. But once again problems came when firms saw the advances made and tried to adapt them for their own products. They designed similar ones but didn't quite get it right. One imitation of the Birmingham design was the Articular Surface Replacement XL Acetabular. At first it seemed to be brilliant and everybody wanted one. One surgeon alone, at a hospital not too far away from here, put in 700 of them. But within two or three years of the product being introduced most of them started coming away. Tiny metal particles were finding their way into the surrounding tissue. That caused a reaction and destroyed tissue, leaving large holes that are difficult to rebuild. Understandably, the patients weren't happy about the situation. At first they tried to sue the surgeons but they couldn't. So they sued the companies instead. DuPuy Orthopaedics currently face thousands of legal cases from people whose hips have fallen out because of a fault in the design of the ASR XL. It's also costing a fortune to put them all right. A primary joint replacement costs about £12,000 privately, including nursing care and the cost of the joint itself. But a revision joint – that is, taking out a failed replacement and putting a new one in – costs around £20,000. Revisions are more technically difficult because a lot of bone has already been removed or damaged, so you need to use a bigger prosthesis. Somebody has to foot the bill for all the hundreds of revisions needed.

I was involved in the development of another hip in the 1990s. We knew that over time the cement we used could cause problems. You clean out the shaft of the thigh bone, fill it with cement and then stick the joint in under pressure until it sets. But the cement can come loose and we were looking for alternative methods of fixing it into the bone. There's a chemical called hydroxyapatite, which is the basic building block of bone. It was discovered that if you sprayed it onto the joint, the bone grows into it when it's packed into the thigh bone, solving the problem of the cement coming loose. Up to this time joints had a rough surface of sprayed on steel bobbles. The bone grew into the little bobbles, interlocked and held. But hydroxyapatite was a far superior solution. A branch of Pfizer asked me to help assess their design. They knew I did lots of hips and asked me to look at their prototype. I thought it was worth a try. It was called the ABG 1. We had ten groups including me, one in France, one in Spain, one in Italy, one in West Germany and one in East Germany – which was difficult because we met every year and he couldn't come because the Russians wouldn't give him a visa. We met at different locations and presented our results to each other. It was all very open and done properly and the results were good. After two years it was released for public use and initially it did very well. But by year five or six problems started emerging. Joints were loosening and coming out. There was a major enquiry and people were threatening to sue. Pfizer asked me to be their expert witness, putting together a report on all the evidence to be used in their defence when the case came to court. I virtually wrote a book on the ABG 1, starting from the genesis of hip joint replacements and going through its entire history. I wrote about the problems with cementing, why hydroxyapatite was beneficial and gave my views about why these joints might have failed. As so often is the case, it was all about the way they were done. Surgeons just weren't being accurate enough. When you put the cup in it has to be at a forty-five degree inclination. If you do it correctly there's more pressure on the outside of the cup and that's where the wearing is. If it's in the right position you get equal wear and the joint remains in place functioning properly for years. Most of the ones we saw failed because of relatively poor surgery. After I retired four of my peers, all working joint replacement surgeons, reviewed the 300 or 400 ABG 1s I put in during that couple of years. Seventy percent were still functioning perfectly well at seventeen years. To put that in perspective, if seven out of ten of any joint lasts seven years that's pretty good going, so I'm happy with that. Although mine did all right I visited several North East hospitals where the results were disastrous. The key was that I'd learned how to fit them properly. I went to Montpelier University twice and stayed with the French surgeon who developed the joint, a lovely man called José Adrey. I watched every detail of his technique because my experience taught me you had to do that. The case was eventually dropped and they couldn't sue Pfizer for negligence. At the end of my career I was using a similar type of joint, although it was a slightly more improved version, the ABG 2. Over the years they got to know where the failures might occur and were able to refine the design. The ABG 1 had a smooth cup with a small hole in the top. The back of a cup was placed in a metal retainer. The engineers believed that any particles of worn plastic would go through the hole and into the metal back of the cup, instead of getting in the tissues, making it safe. As it turned out that wasn't a good idea because more plastic was worn off, especially if the cup wasn't in precisely the right position. Everything that moves wears and they learned that continuous tiny movements wore off particles of plastic from the front and back of the cup. So they modified the fixation of the cup slightly and it seems to have solved the problem. The ABG 2 was in use for a while but now it's gone.

The science has to advance all the time, but there are proper ways to do things. First of all you do extensive *in vitro* tests using machines. If you can manipulate a knee joint twenty million times in test conditions and there's no wear on it, it's looking good. But then you have to test it on groups of real people. And crucially, you have to train people to do it properly. You can't just give it to one surgeon. He could do thousands of them successfully and then other people read about it and decide they'll have a go. But if the first surgeon is a perfectionist and the ones who follow have never actually been to see him, that can create problems. He's done them all his own way, but everybody else tries to modify the procedure and the joint ends up falling to pieces. My guiding principle has always been that if someone develops something that looks promising, go and see it for yourself. I learnt this from Sir John Charnley. In those days, you weren't allowed to buy a Charnley hip joint unless you'd been properly trained in how to put it in. That's the way it should be. That was also the advice I gave Derek McMinn when he was developing Birmingham Hip Resurfacing. I told him to get five or ten groups of surgeons at five or ten different centres to do fifty each and then to watch them for two years, because if they're going to fail quickly, they go within that timeframe. If they all get the same result at the end of the trial then it can be released for use on the general public. That seems to be happening more and more now, where companies get several centres together to compare results. But others still haven't learned their lesson. They're still giving them to just one or two surgeons and the rest of the world only read about it in the media. Every time some new "miracle op" was reported in the press I'd get a queue of patients who wanted one. They had read that it would allow them to leave hospital after two days and be back at work in six weeks. My clinic the following week would be taken up telling people like Mr Jones, who's seventy-eight, why he doesn't need one. I'd explain that we knew the hips we already had would last him until the end of his life anyway – and we're not at all sure about all the problems the new joint would bring. Ultimately, though, if people want something and they can afford it, they'll go away and find somebody else who will do it. And there are always people out there who will do it for the money, whether it's in the patient's best interests or not. I've been involved in a few cases around the country where surgeons have carried out procedures they didn't have the necessary experience for, and they've crippled people.

The more operations you do the more expertise you gain and the more people get to hear about you. When problems started to come to light with certain hips, the Medicines and Healthcare Products Regulatory Agency asked me to look into it. Another time the Medical Defence Union asked me to examine hips in an area of the country where there'd been lots of problems. I'd sometimes look at the cases and say, "Well, the surgeon shouldn't really have done that." But other times I would find myself saying, "There but for the grace of God go I."

Throughout most of my surgical career, I used monoblock joints, meaning the stem is all in one piece. As the years went on they started producing replacements with variable lengths that could be adapted to fit patients better. But the problem is that once you put a head onto a metal projection you get fretting and corrosion and again, metal particles came come away and get into the surrounding tissues, causing serious damage.

You've got to look at each development so carefully. If I didn't think a new joint was based on good mechanical principles I wouldn't use it. Then you can sit back smugly years later and say "I told you so" when it goes wrong! Or if I saw a joint I wasn't entirely sure about, I might try one or two to see how they work. There is a huge responsibility on the surgeon. But it's the duty of the manufacturer to do all the laboratory and clinical testing on it before they release the joint or even let the public know about it. You can't just produce something and rush to get it on the shelves as quickly as possible for half the price of everything else on the market. Yes, you'll start a stampede of people wanting to give it a go. But I can tell you that years of experience proves it's just not the way to do it.

16

Joint Responsibility

I think people have learnt their lesson now. The profession is once again coming round to the way we used to do things and an insistence that patients have to be followed up for life. The biggest single development in this respect has been the establishment of the National Joint Registry.

The disastrous copy Charnley prostheses produced after the patent expired in the 1990s increased the belief among orthopaedics experts that something must be done to regulate the field. Thousands of sub-standard hips had been fitted to patients around the world and it was causing enormous problems. We lobbied the government on the issue and the result was the registry, which began in 2003. Initially it only covered hips and knees because they were the most common operations, with 60,000 of each carried out every year in this country alone. Every time a surgeon carried out a joint replacement they were asked to fill in a form stating what he's put in and how he's performed the procedure. Then the patient fills in another form saying how they're doing afterwards.

I was a founder member of the National Joint Registry Committee. In addition, every area of the country had its own regional representative, and I was the North East Clinical Director. My role involved going to hospitals and trying to ensure everyone complied with the new system. It wasn't a legal obligation at the time, but it would only work if everyone did it, so we impressed on them the importance of doing so. Some surgeons were worried their work coming under public scrutiny and resisted. I remember joking, "Would you ask a surgeon to operate on one of your patients if you didn't know what his results were like?" It was hard work, going round like a travelling salesman, but eventually the numbers started to come in and people realised what the benefits were.

I also was medical secretary of the Nuffield Doctors' Committee at that time. I told the hospital that if doctors refused to comply with the register I didn't think they should be given rights to operate there. They didn't like that idea. But I believed it was the right thing to do. In the end the private hospitals were the first ones to be fully compliant, filling in every detail.

Once the system was underway we were getting reports on thousands of hips a year and held an annual meeting in London to examine the results. We could see how many of each joint had been used and what their comparative success rates were. We could say the Charnley's doing brilliantly, the Exeter's doing very well, but this one's not so good and this other one's a disaster.

After I retired from James Cook I continued going round nine North East hospitals to monitor what they were doing and advise them. Another advantage having had so many trainees go through the hospital and then going on to work throughout the north was that I knew just about everybody in the region. When I wanted to talk to them about the register they couldn't just say they didn't have time to see me. When I rang I would hear, "Oh hello, Mr A! When would you like to come?" So I had no trouble at all. When I went to the meetings in London, everyone else would be complaining that people couldn't be bothered to see them. For that reason we were one of the first regions to really take off in terms of our compliance with the National Joint Registry. The annual meeting meant getting up 5am, catching the 6.30am train down of London and sitting in a meeting all day before coming home back that night. The last two times I went I stayed over the night before. But as I got on a bit I wasn't quite mobile enough and I gave it up in 2012. I said, "I've had enough guys, get some new blood in."

The register now covers hips, knees, shoulders, elbows and ankles, things I was doing experimentally up here in the 1970s and 80s. Joint replacement started off in hips but over the years, as prosthetic knee joints developed and the technology improved, the number of knees has caught up with the number of hips. It used to be perhaps 40,000 hips to 25,000 knees, but it's about equal now. There are about 60,000 of each every year and they're all being entered into the National Joint Register, together with all those other joint operations. Because we've been doing them so long and now analyse the data, we know what you should expect if they're done properly. If I was still operating and replaced a knee joint I would have to be able to tell the patient it has a ninety-five per cent chance of lasting ten years. A hip must have a ninety-five per cent chance of lasting fifteen years. The fact that the patient is told how long it should last means that if it fails within three years, they know something's not right. Either they've knocked it about and gone paragliding, high-jumping or marathon running, or it's faulty or hasn't been put in correctly. I saw one patient of forty-five boasting on TV that he was back fell running within a year of having his new hip fitted. That's exactly what you tell people not to do. You don't want artificial joints to suffer repeated impact loading such as running and jumping.

We now know that Charnley joints and some of the others will last for twenty-to-thirty years, so you don't need to see patients for a follow-up every year, you can make it year one, year two, year five, year seven and then every three years after that. That's quite acceptable with an established joint, but you can't do that with a new one that's only been on the market for a couple of years. The metal-on-metal joints should be followed up every year because of the serious problems they're causing. That recommendation has gone to the Government from the British Orthopaedic Association. We've told them what we think should be followed up and why, and someone will have to find the money to do it. It's not as though an x-ray of a hip joint every couple of years costs that much. We've suggested the insurance companies should pay for private patients and the NHS pay for its own patients. Currently, if you have a private hip or knee replacement at the Nuffield, the private insurance companies will only pay for one follow up. They'll see you maybe six weeks, six months or a year later, and then that's it, goodbye. If you get a problem you'll have to pay again for an x-ray and a visit to the specialist.

The technology continues to develop, with mixed results. They've been through metal-on-metal resurfacing and then large metal-on-metal heads like a tennis ball on a stem, which are also failing. In some ways it's come round in a full circle. Surgeons are putting hips back in with cement and hydroxyapatite, although they're using ceramic instead of plastic now. But if something doesn't look right with a particular prosthesis that comes onto the market we're in a much better position to identify the issue as soon as things begin to go wrong. That's the great advantage that's come out of the National Joint Registry. It's been a giant step forward and has improved standards dramatically.

17

Doc Holidays

There's nothing quite like the taste of that first gin and tonic on the plane as you set off on a well-earned holiday. Lying back and watching the land disappear away below you is one of life's great pleasures. It was usually a last dash panic to get away on time after finishing work and Freda was always complaining because I was so disorganised. We loved to stay in the El Fuerte hotel, right in the centre of Marbella and just a short walk up to the square where the church is. It's a lovely place, a real old fashioned, traditional Spanish town. We discovered the hotel completely by accident. I stayed there when I was asked to chair a meeting on knee replacements by one of the manufacturers. They often choose the surgeons who did the most operations to speak at these events. In return they offered you free or reduced airfare and accommodation – which is fair enough. You paid a nominal sum if you were invited to bring your wife, but you were staying in a double room anyway so it was no skin off their nose. Some people really took advantage of such generosity and went all round the world at the companies' expense. I was watching television one night when I saw a train full of consultants going to Venice on the Orient Express – including one of ours! That sort of thing isn't allowed anymore, and quite rightly so. You now have to declare each year any gifts you've accepted from drug or medical equipment firms. We liked the El Fuerte so much that we started visiting regularly. We loved to go in May because it coincided with the First

Communion celebrations at the church in the square and it was always such a joyful and beautiful occasion. Then we went again in September, when it was quiet and peaceful, after the kids had gone back to school. The hotel knew us and we stayed in the same room every time, on the top floor with a stunning sea view balcony. We could walk straight out of the front door and stroll into the village in a few minutes. We loved Spain.

As well as those two weeks in the sun we'd go to Paris for a few days in July and maybe again in November. We always flew out from Newcastle on July 13th and stayed for Bastille Day, which was terrific, and the next day was Freda's birthday. Freda and I loved the atmosphere and vibrancy of Paris, especially at night. We would just drift around the streets, taking in the sights and eating outside cosy bistros. We stayed in different places. We tried the very best, including Margaret Thatcher's favourite Hôtel de Crillon, in the Place de la Concorde, and we once had a bargain break at The Ritz, which was the headquarters of the SS during the war. It's a magnificent building, down one of the side streets just off the Champs-Elysées. Although it was a wonderful experience we felt very much like the poor folks staying there, with all the wealth and opulence all around us. Usually, though, we'd book into a little *pension*, staying in a tiny little room you couldn't swing a cat in. Often you couldn't even open the bathroom door outwards because the rooms were so small. Unfortunately, we're not able to go abroad anymore. I'm quite fragile from the waist downwards and also developed diabetes two years before I retired. I had it for a long time before it was diagnosed. One night I was lying in bed and I couldn't feel my feet.

"Have I got my socks on?" I asked Freda. Every man's done that at some time, usually when he's had a few too many drinks – but this night I hadn't. Eventually I went to see a colleague, who examined me and said I was a hypochondriac. During my last six months of work, when I went back to help them get the link up with the Friarage Hospital in Northallerton going, I started really struggling. I was exhausted for no reason and in the last week before I finally retired I went to my GP to have some blood tests. After my last day at work we went off to Paris for a relaxing weekend. While I was away I received a phone call from the surgery. They didn't want me to panic but told me to go to see them when I got back on Monday morning. My blood sugar levels showed I had neuropathy, damage to the nerves, which was causing the numbness. They couldn't do anything about it and it's just become progressively worse. It's gone right up my legs now and I don't feel much at all. You have a sense called proprioception, the messages your nerves send your brain to tell it you where your fingers are. When the neuropathy reaches your legs you can't tell where you're putting your feet and so I fall over, which is very embarrassing.

I also developed arthritis in my hip in about 2002. One of my trainees, Ananda Nanu, said I was walking with external rotation of my right leg and had arthritis in my hip. "Good lad," I thought. "You'll do well." And he has done well. Next year he's president of the British Orthopaedic Association. He was with us as a trainee, got a consultant's job in Sunderland now he's a Professor. It always gives me a great sense of pride when lads I've taught do well.

I can't run these days, I have arthritis in my legs and if I walk fifty metres I take a stick. But you just get on with it. I noticed it more after I retired. I fell off my bike when a Mini came across and I moved in and hit the kerb, hurting my knee. I couldn't straighten it and deep down I knew I'd torn a cartilage, but I was hoping against hope that I hadn't. I rang Tony Hoy, who I'd appointed as knee surgeon. I was hoping he'd give me an injection. But when I went to see him he delivered the bad news I was fearing.

"You know that an injection isn't going to help, don't you?" he said.

"I know," I replied glumly.

I was in the next morning, scoped at seven o'clock and back home at noon. I was on my bike again and going to the gym within three weeks. But now, sadly, the other knee has started playing up.

Between the arthritis and the neuropathy I'm not as steady on my feet as I'd like to be. On our last trip to Paris we were on our way to a restaurant we liked and I fell over while we were coming up from the Metro. It frightened Freda. She was worried that if anything happened to me when we were overseas she wouldn't know what to do. I would love to go back to Marbella and Paris but I'd struggle now. I've just got to accept that those wonderful days are behind me.

18

Pain in Spain

The only time we went on holiday more than our usual week it very nearly ended in tragedy. It was 2002 and for some reason we decided to go to Spain for a fortnight. At the end of the first week we went out for a meal with a gang of friends from Teesside. There was the dentist, Dave Moore, Eric McMordie, the former Boro and Northern Ireland footballer, and Foster Garton, who built Tennis World in Middlesbrough. I got to know Foss after I treated him for a bad back. They carried him off a plane and brought him to see me and I gave him an injection and got him back on his feet. He thought I was marvellous and we've been firm friends ever since. He and his pals were all great golfers and tried to persuade me to play. But quite honestly, I just haven't got the patience. They'd invite me for a game at two o'clock on a Thursday afternoon and I'd turn up ten minutes late because I'd be finishing off a session in theatre. Despite the validity of my excuse, they didn't like that at all. In the end I thought, "Sod them!" – and I've never played since. I've got a magnificent set of Callaghan carbon fibre clubs in the garage that I'm going to give to my son Ben because he's a keen golfer and is big and powerful. Ben and I used to play nine holes for money on holiday in Spain when he'd just taken up the game as a young teenager. Needless to say, he always won. People would tell him, "Ben, you should be saving your pocket money for Spain" and he'd say, "No need, I'll just win it off Dad when we get there!" Foss had a villa in Spain and went over often and we would meet up and socialise together. When we got home that night Freda didn't feel very well and started to be sick. As time went on she got worse and worse. By the following day she was severely dehydrated, in pain and badly swollen. I called the doctor who was attached to the hotel. He was Spanish but had done part of his training in Manchester. He examined her and said she needed to come into hospital. She was admitted to a private clinic a few doors down from the hotel. They looked after her well there, but her condition didn't improve and the swelling to her abdomen was getting bigger and bigger. The doctor insisted it was nothing more than "holiday tummy". After three or four days, she still wasn't getting any better. I told him I was an orthopaedic surgeon, but even I could tell him it definitely was not gastroenteritis. By this time she was becoming quite ill. I rang the insurance company and told them I was concerned and wanted to get her home. They offered to med-evac her home within forty-eight hours. I told them that would be too late, she would be dead by them. The situation really was that grave. There was a plane leaving the next morning. Although she wasn't really fit to fly, I persuaded the doctors to sign a certificate saying she was. When we reached the airport the next day, Freda couldn't walk. I had to drag her out of the taxi and into the terminal. The queues for our flight stretched all the way out of the building. I went to the desk and pleaded with them.

"My wife is really quite ill and she can't stand in this queue," I said. They said I could queue for her but they wouldn't let us have a wheelchair until we were through security. Freda needed to lie down. I asked the hostess and she said the only place was the first class lounge. I paid the fee and we went in. It was empty and there was a sofa, so I plumped up the cushions up and got her comfortable. Who should walk in just then, but Cilla Black and Dale Winton! I could see them looking over and thinking, "Look at that, another drunken Brit abroad!" I somehow got Freda onto the plane they gave us an easy access seat. I was terrified. It was the worst flight of my life. I was once in an aircraft that was forced to make an emergency landing coming into Masirah Island, off the coast of Oman. I was frightened for my own life that night, but I was far more frightened now of losing my wife. She couldn't eat or drink and was really poorly. I'd rung one of my mates at the hospital, a general surgeon.

I said I thought she probably had a perforation and arranged for her to come straight in. We landed at Teesside and my son Matthew was waiting for us. At first we went to the Nuffield but she was sent straight to James Cook in an ambulance while I followed behind. It was a traumatic journey for me, bringing painful memories flooding back. In 1967, when I was stationed at RAF Cosford, I'd followed an ambulance in the middle of the night from hospital in Wolverhampton to a special baby unit in Birmingham. It was carrying my baby Thomas, who had been injured at birth and later died. Here I was again, now following an ambulance that was rushing my dangerously ill wife to an awaiting emergency team. After we arrived they took some scans but she wasn't well enough to operate on that night. Instead they booked her in for surgery the following morning. Then came a shattering blow. The tests showed she had suffered a massive haemorrhage in her stomach. It had killed part of her bowel off and they needed to remove it. When your stomach is inflamed or you have peritonitis, your diaphragm, which should move up and down when you breathe, is splinted. You can't breathe properly and get double pneumonia, which is what had happened to Freda. The surgeon didn't try to hide the severity of the situation from me. He told me there was a very good chance Freda would die on the operating table.

They took her to theatre first thing the next morning and she was in there for what seemed like an age. She lost about eight-feet of bowel and was taken to intensive care. She couldn't talk and had a tube down her. The family were there every day. It was an incredibly difficult time for all of us. The first couple of weeks was desperately worrying. I was still working and the staff were very kind and understanding. Everybody knew me when I went in to visit. I had time off when I needed it but when she was in intensive care there was no point in sitting around all day waiting. I continued working just along the corridor whenever I could.

Eventually they took the tube out of her and told us she wouldn't be able to talk for a couple of days. Freda communicated by writing messages on pieces of paper. The first words she wrote?

"I really liked that purple anorak I saw in Escada..."

Matthew got straight on the phone, rang up Corte Ingles, the big department store in Marbella, and asked to be put through to the Escada counter. He told them his mother had seen a lilac-coloured ladies' sports anorak and asked if it was still available. It was. He ordered it and it arrived a couple of days afterwards.

When she contracted the antibiotic-resistant infection MRSA I said there was no point keeping her in hospital any longer. Instead she came home and I injected her every night with intravenous antibiotics.

"If I wanted to get rid of you I could slip you a Micky Finn," I joked. Fortunately we could laugh about it by this stage, but we'd all been very shaken and upset by what had happened. It took Freda two years to get back to normal. She'd been very, very ill. Later she told us she could remember lying in a room and hearing a voice in the corner saying, "You can come now if you want, Freda, we're ready for you." Fortunately, her time wasn't up. But she was very emotional as she continued on the long road to recovery. She couldn't go into the body of the church because if people she knew asked how she was she would break down in tears. So we'd stand behind the glass partition at the back of the Holy Name.

Lying unconscious in intensive care had caused Freda to lose the hair on the back of her head from the pressure on it. Ever since we were students she'd always gone to London regularly to have her hair done by John Frieda. He was married to the singer, Lulu. In a strange twist of fate Lulu was on in Scarborough when we went there for our honeymoon in 1966. That night she had climbed out of a taxi and ran past us shouting, "Hi!" Years later we found ourselves chatting away in the salon as her husband cut my wife's hair. Freda couldn't face going back to John Frieda after losing her hair. She said she would have felt too emotional.

"I wouldn't mind trying Nicky Clark," she said. So I rang up and he offered me an urgent appointment for a cut and blow for £500 – and that was 2002 prices! But if that was what Freda wanted it was what Freda would get and I made an appointment – only for her to change her mind!

We celebrated our Golden Wedding anniversary on April 2nd 2016 and we knew each other for six years before we married. People ask me how I can still remember the date we first went out together, May 9th 1959, when we went to see *The Nun's Story*. Well, I just do. You remember things that mean a lot to you. I remember it every year and send Freda a card saying how many years it's been since that first date. It was a major milestone in my life. We've been together for almost six decades and I've never looked back for a single moment.

19

A Family Home

We love having a houseful of children. Sometimes we might have eight here for a weekend and they just kip down anywhere they can. That's why we don't have one of these little dinky-do, neat and tidy houses. Freda has always said, "It's not a house, it's a home." They get free reign to run about all over the place and enjoy it. Family's been hugely important to us, although for most of our fifty years together I was never in. Freda never knew when to cook a meal and she'd often end up out in the kitchen getting something ready for me at ten o'clock at night. That's just how it was. I needed unfailing support in the job I was in and Freda was always there for me. Being a teacher she was great with kids and she brought our children up. I feel embarrassed when I see what my sons do in the house now and the time they spend with their children. I was never around. I worked all week, then on Saturdays I'd do private jobs at the Nuffield and on Sundays I might do some medico-legal work. We enjoyed family holidays, to Spain, Portugal and staying in static caravans near Cannes, and had wonderful times together. But when we were at home I was invariably working.

Richard was born in 1967. A year later, we had another son, Thomas Martin. Tragically, he sustained an injury at birth and died at just four months old. That was an incredibly difficult time for both of us, but especially for Freda. I was on duty at the hospital one night and when I came in I noticed the house was unusually quiet. "The kids are normally up at this time," I thought. When

I went upstairs Freda was asleep and Thomas was lying in the cot, cold and blue. Freda suffered very badly and there was no help available for people in those days, it was just considered hard luck. It hit me hard as well. As a doctor, when death confronts you like that, you know that these things happen all the time. It does, you know. People die. But when it's your own it's very different, and I was extremely upset. Less than a year later, in 1969, we had Matthew. Rachael came next, so we had three boys and a girl, and then Eddie. After that there was a ten-year gap. It looked like our little family was complete. But in 1984, after I had the car accident, we went away to Spain while I recovered. Ben was born nine months later.

All the children went to St Edward's Primary School, behind the Holy Name of Mary Church. Richard was naturally bright and didn't need private education. Besides, I couldn't afford it when he was growing up. He studied Accountancy at the London School of Economics and later moved into banking and now mortgages. Richard's wife is Ruth and they have two children, Eve and Charlie. The day Eve was born I was at a hip joint meeting at Chatsworth House. It was a cold, frosty November morning and I smoked then. Everybody smoked when I was younger. If you watch old films they've all got fags in their hands. I gave it up many years ago, thankfully. I remember an old commander in the RAF saying, "Anderson, the life you lead, you'll be dead by the time you're forty." As well as smoking I was also drinking a lot, keeping up with the guys from the fighter squadrons. During a break at Chatsworth I came outside for a cigarette and while I was strolling around the gardens my phone rang. It was Rich.

"Dad," he said. "We've just had a little girl." I was overjoyed.

When Matthew reached secondary school age we decided he needed some extra help. Matthew was very technically minded. At the age of twelve he was taking washing machines apart and putting them back together again. We took the decision not to send him to the local school and I wanted to him to go to Ampleforth, but Freda's a mother and didn't want him too far away from her apron strings. Instead we sent him to Yarm School. He didn't want to stay there for the sixth form and went to Prior Pursglove Sixth Form, at Guisborough, which he enjoyed. After that he did a Mechanical

Engineering degree in London. He can do anything he wants to. He works very hard as an engineer for the Weir Group, specialising in bearings for nuclear plants. Nuclear reactors need water to keep them cool, otherwise they explode. When one of them starts to fail he goes out to sort it, which means travelling all over the world. He also has a little boy, Oliver, who is twelve and lives with his mum. Ollie is an enthusiastic skater and does all kinds of tricks. He was number one in the North East for his age group, but unfortunately, he had a nasty break of his right ankle and was out of action for a long time.

Our next child is our only daughter, Rachael. She went to Teesside High girls' school after primary school, then went off to London and did a degree in French and Literature. She worked as an interpreter in Hong Kong for a few months, then came back and married Francis Martin, who is the son of two Middlesbrough teachers, at the Sacred Heart Church. They have three children, Max, who's thirteen, Xavier, who's ten, and Mary, who's nine. They're lovely kids and I get to spend a lot of time with them because they're all very sporty. Max and Xavier are ace footballers and Xavier's had a contract with York City from the age of eight. I go down to watch him at the weekends.

A couple of years after Rachael, Edward came along. He also went to Yarm School after primary school and he did very well. After studying Law in Manchester, he decided to specialise in European Law. Private school fees had already cost me an arm and a leg and Eddie's decision meant yet more expense for me because I had to pay for him to do his Masters in Bruges! After that, the big London firms just jumped on him. Normally it's a three-day interview to get a job. He put his application in and they offered him the job on the spot. What's more, thank God, they paid for him for the last six months of his course, which saved me a bit of money and gave him some extra cash to spend. We loved going to Bruges to visit him. We'd go through the Channel Tunnel and spend a couple of nights in Bruges, which is a lovely city. Eddie and his wife Kiki live in London, where he's now a senior lawyer. They have three children, Joseph, Sophie and Rosa.

Then, when I was well into my forties, we had Ben, our baby. He went to Yarm School. From the age of about fourteen Ben surfed at Saltburn. Rach and her husband, Francis, lived in Barbados for two years just after they got married and Ben went there every school holiday to perfect his surfing skills. After school he had a few gap years, taking the chance to travel all round the world, including Australia and Thailand. He's been just about everywhere. Eventually he came back and said, "I think I'll start again." So he got the equivalent of A levels and studied physiotherapy in Plymouth. Shortly after he qualified the NHS stopped offering training posts. He decided physiotherapy was a bit of a dead end because there weren't the jobs available. He's always been in good shape so he took up fitness training and worked in gyms in London and all over the North East. He was with all the big firms, including Bannatynes and David Lloyd. Then he found out about a run-down ladies' gym in Northallerton. The owner was a property developer and was too busy with that side of his business and had neglected the gym. He offered Ben the chance to rent it for three years and see if he could get it off the ground, with the opportunity to buy if after that. He's working really hard to make a success of it. He's trebled the attendance levels and does as much advertising as he can. Ben married Kat in the summer and they live at Norton. He had a relationship before that and has a son, Louis, who's very much part of the gang and we see him every week. We still see his mam, Laura, as well, because it was an amicable separation and she's also very much part of the family. Louis gave us all a terrible scare when he got a particularly nasty form cancer of childhood cancer. It was a neuroblastoma, a cancer of the sympathetic nerves at the back of your abdomen. Of those who get it, seventy-two per cent die in the first two years. Louis was pale, tired and lethargic. He didn't want to play with the other kids and was listless and whiny. Laura took him to the doctor's over and over again but kept being told it was nothing serious. I advised her to take him to the Casualty Department at Durham. At least he would see a specialist doctor. But even then they just said he had constipation. One week they came here and he really was ill. It was quite clear there was something very wrong and I decided I had to do something. I rang my mate Geoff Wyatt, the paediatrician at James Cook.

"It's my grandson, Geoff," I said. "He's very ill and I think he's going to die in the next fortnight if somebody doesn't find out what's wrong."

He agreed to see him the next day. At last we'd found someone who realised how serious things were. He immediately got him into the Oncology Unit at Newcastle, where they discovered an enormous tumour. For two or three years he was very ill. He spent a lot of time in the RVI at Newcastle and underwent chemotherapy, radiotherapy and major surgery, losing a kidney and the adrenal glands that the cancer had invaded. They put him on steroids, which had unfortunate side-effects, including making him aggressive towards his cousins.

One of the worst things was seeing the children he was being treated alongside all dying, one by one. We all wondered whether Louis would be next. That was a very sad time for us. I was up and down to Newcastle a lot to give him support, and so was Ben. Then the oncologist told us about a new antibody treatment that actually targeted the cancer cells and killed them off. They couldn't get a licence for it in England at that time and so they told us we'd have to wait. It had to be given when the child's immune system has been lowered, or the body's defences would attack the antibody and destroy it. Shortly after his last chemotherapy session, when his immune system was at its lowest, the licence was issued and Louis was given it straight away. He was quite ill again after that but kids are remarkably resilient. Louis is nearly ten now and he's cured. They check him up once a year but now he's come this far I know he'll be all right. He's captain of Sacriston Juniors in Durham and is in the North East Football Academy. They won a trophy that's almost as big as him in a competition last year. He's quite a character. He comes over and stays with us once every couple of weeks when all the other kids come. I sometimes look at photographs from that time when he was really ill now and I can't believe it's our Louis in them.

We only see Eddie and his family twice a year but the others are here together an awful lot. Richard's two kids are getting a bit older now. Eve is sixteen and she won't want to be with little kids for much longer. She's so much older than the other grandchildren at the house and the little girls have always loved her and looked up to her. Whenever they get together they all get made up and have their nails painted. We've put nets and hoops up in the garden and they're always out playing basketball or football, or they're upstairs playing on Xboxes, although we try to discourage them from being on them too much. The rule is that when we go out anywhere they turn them off. As they get out the car I say, "Right guys, the electronics please!" All the phones are switched off and left in the car. If you don't do that they'll spend hour after hour on them. It ruins conversation and they'll never learn to spell and write properly. So at least when we go out anywhere we all talk to each other. Sometimes as soon as they get here I say, "Right, no electronics for an hour, come on, we'll sit and have a chat." Then they all talk. Otherwise they'll mumble at you and look at their messages all night. Of course, if I'd had all those gadgets in my day, I'd probably have been playing games as they do. Maybe I wouldn't have spent my time reading about planes and anaesthesia and medical history, and been wouldn't have inspired to take the path in my life that I did.

Towards the end of my career, we'd just had another grandchild when I received a call from the girl in the Trust press office.

"Congratulations," she said.

"Yes, it's great news," I said. "Just what I wanted, a granddaughter."

"No, not that," she said. "You've been awarded a CBE for services to medicine."

I thought it was a joke. Everybody gets an OBE, even the chief executive from James Cook, Bill Murray, had got one! But a CBE was a bit special. I couldn't settle that night and stayed up until midnight, when *The Times* is published online. I scoured through the whole list of showbiz stars and lollipop ladies until I got to the CBEs – and there I was. I couldn't believe it. I was thrilled to bits.

Freda wouldn't come to Buckingham Palace.

"You spent all your life working and didn't see much of the kids," she said. "Take the three boys with you instead."

Ben was away in Australia so Richard, Matthew and Eddie came and we all thoroughly enjoyed the experience.

I sat next to Mrs Bucket from TV's *Keeping Up Appearances*, the actress Patricia Routledge, who was being made a Dame the same day. She was a knockout. She wouldn't shut up – just like her TV character! There was a band out in the hall and, I have to admit, they were completely out of tune and ruining everything they played. Nobody else mentioned it, but she was laughing and joking.

"For God's sake," I said. "You'll end up in the Bloody Tower if you go on like this."

She was fascinated by my profession.

"How many guineas do you charge for a new knee joint?" she asked.

"We don't do it in guineas these days," I replied. "But if you need me, you can always come and find me up in Teesside."

The Queen was lovely. It was at the time when the late Queen Mother was having trouble with her hips.

"My mother could do with seeing you!" the Queen told me.

People pulled my leg no end about the honour and I was given the nickname "Top Doc". I had to take my medal to the hospital and show them and people even stopped me in the car park to congratulate me. But if I needed bringing back down to earth, a hospital was the perfect place to be. I went to Northallerton to do a theatre list and they cut a piece of silver paper out and wrote "CBeebies" on it!

When I went to Buckingham Palace I was told, "We don't often give CBEs to doctors, you must have done something really special. Normally you have to discover DNA because that's how Watson and Crick got theirs!"

It was nice to hear, but I gave them an honest reply.

"I didn't do anything special at all," I said. "I just did my job."

Receiving the CBE was a great honour and I'm still very proud of it. But it wasn't something I ever expected. Being able to serve the people of my hometown in the way I did was a wonderful privilege. For me, it was never about money, recognition or status in society. It would be very hard to beat the feeling of seeing the happiness that a new hip or knee joint gave my patients and the transformation in their lives that followed. That's all the reward I could ever ask for.

Printed in Great Britain
by Amazon